The Dao Of
Increasing
Longevity And
Conserving
One's Life

The Dao Of Increasing Longevity And Conserving One's Life

A Handbook Of Traditional Chinese Geriatrics And Chinese Herbal Patent Medicines

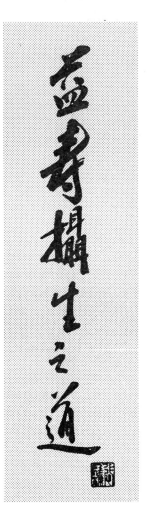

by
Anna Lin
&
Bob Flaws

Blue Poppy Press

Published by:

BLUE POPPY PRESS
1775 LINDEN AVE.
BOULDER, CO 80304

FIRST EDITION
JUNE 1991

ISBN 0-936185-24-4

Distributors

AcuMedic CENTRE
101-105 CAMDEN HIGH STREET
LONDON NW1 7JN
Tel: 0171-388 5783/6704
Catalogue on Request

Printed at Westview Press, Boulder, CO

This book is printed on archive quality, acid free, recycled paper.

Calligraphies on the cover, pages xvi, 24, 78, and 148 by Zhang Ting-liang.

Calligraphy on facing page by Xing Kong, Abbot of the Cold Mountain Monastery, Zhejiang Province.

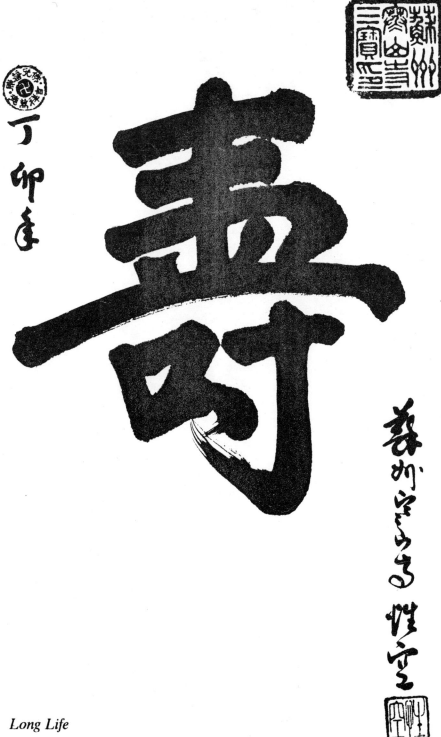

Long Life

Foreword

This book is based on a Chinese text entitled *Lao Ren Bao Jian Zhong Cheng Yao (Chinese Herbal Patent Medicines for Protecting the Health of the Elderly)* compiled by Shen Lian-sheng and Li Guo-qing and published by the People's Hygiene Press in Beijing in 1984. It is not a complete translation. Much of the descriptions of the individual Chinese patent medicines included in the original have already been published in English, such as the functions of each individual ingredient in each prescription. Therefore, we have limited ourselves to merely listing the ingredients of each medicine described and each medicine's indications. We have also for the most part, not included those Chinese patent medicines which are currently not available in the United States.

In preparing this book, we queried several distributors of Chinese patent medicines here in the United States as to which of the medicines included in the original they carried. Only two distributors replied, Mayway Trading Corporation of San Francisco and Nuherbs Company of Oakland, CA. We have noted after each medicine which of these two distributors carries it and these two companies' addresses are given in an appendix. We did not feel it would be fair to practitioners to discuss alot of patent medicines not available to them in their practice. Some of the medicines discussed which are not available as patents are available as powdered extracts. In a very few instances we have discussed formulas which, although not available in prepared form, may be given as decoctions made from bulk dispensed herbs. These have been included because they treat an important pattern covering a commonly encountered geriatric disease.

We have also taken the liberty to add material to this text taken from other, already available, English language books on Chinese patent medicines. These sources include *Chinese Herbal Patent Formulas, A Practical Guide* by Jake Fratkin, Institute for Traditional Medicine, Portland, OR; *Outline Guide to Chinese Herbal Patent Medicines in Pill Form* by Margaret A. Naeser, Boston Chinese Medicine, Boston, MA; and *Clinical Handbook of Chinese Prepared Medicines* by Chun-han Zhu, Paradigm Publications, Brookline, MA. We refer the interested reader looking for more detailed explanations of individual medicines to these three books. Although they do not discuss all the medicines included in this book, they do cover a great many of them. In addition, these books include other patent medicines not contained herein which may also be appropriate for the treatment of various conditions discussed in this book. In this text we simply refer to these books by their authors' names.

Because Blue Poppy Press as yet does not have the software to print Chinese characters nor the funds to have these professionally typeset, the identification of the medicinal ingredients in the patent medicines described herein has been given in Latinate pharmacological nomenclature. Our sources for identification were Bensky & Gamble's *Chinese Herbal Medicine: Materia Medica*, Eastland Press, Seattle, WA; Cloudburst Press' *A Barefoot Doctor's Manual*, Mayne Isle & Seattle; Hong-yen Hsu's *Oriental Materia Medica, A Concise Guide*, OHAI Press, Long Beach, CA; and Southern Materials Center's *Chinese Materia Medica,* Vol. 1-6, Taipei, ROC. However, we have changed the word order of some of our identifications as compared to that of our sources. Most of the medicinals included in this book are derived from plant sources.

Therefore, we have placed any modifying adjectives relating to special methods of preparation of that part of the plant in question directly after the noun identifying the plant part as it would be in Latin. For instance, fresh ginger is identified herein as Rhizoma Recens Zingiberis or fresh rhizome of ginger as opposed to Rhizoma Zingiberis Recentis in which case the Recentis may be confused as the second part of the binomial taxonomy.

Readers familiar with other of Blue Poppy Press' books on Chinese medicine will note that in this book we have begun to shift our translational terminology towards that proposed by Nigel Wiseman in *Glossary of Chinese Medical Terms* published by Paradigm Publications, Brookline, MA. As translators of Chinese medicine into English, we substantially agree with Mr. Wiseman in his introduction to that glossary regarding the issues and problems of such an endeavor. It will take us at Blue Poppy Press some time, however, to fully implement Mr. Wiseman's recommendations. Also readers will note that we have begun to decapitalize technical Chinese medical terms translated into English. We believe Western professional practitioners of Chinese medicine are by now sophisticated enough to be able to read technical Chinese medical literature and understand its technical terminology as defined in Chinese medicine without recourse to archaic and inconsistent capitalization.

Beyond these technical issues in the preparation of this book, we have selected this book for publication as part of our on-going attempt to provide clinical manuals for the various specialties within Traditional Chinese Medicine or TCM. Geriatrics is one such specialty which as yet has received little or no attention in the English TCM literature. Because more and more people are living longer and longer, we believe attention to this specialty is due. Further, we believe that

Chinese medicine with its emphasis on prevention and longevity has something unique to contribute to geriatrics worldwide. Its theory of aging and its identification and use of supplementary medicinals supply something that is lacking in modern Western medicine.

Most geriatric conditions are due to emptiness and decline of righteous qi and yin substance, such as blood and *jing*. To an extent, this decline and exhaustion is not really reversible. Its progression is inevitable and inexorable. Therefore, most geriatric conditions are chronic and only remediable within limitation. Medicines, and especially tonics for the supplementation of such emptiness and weakness need to be taken regularly over a long period of time. Strength of individual doses in such cases is less important than the regularity of continued small doses. Patent medicines lend themselves to this need. They are easy to take and, therefore, patients are willing to take them over prolonged periods of time. We feel that, because the Chinese original from which we worked specifically addresses geriatric problems through the prescription of such patent medicines, TCM clinicians treating the elderly will find this book particularly useful and easy to use.

This book is meant as a professional text and not as a layperson's guide. It is offered as a professional clinical manual and also as a textbook on geriatrics for use in schools and colleges of TCM wishing to include this specialty in their curriculum. Lay readers interested in availing themselves of the benefits of the medicines described in this book are advised to seek out a professional practitioner of Chinese medicine. The medicines described herein are not panaceas. Like any medication, they have their indications and contraindications. When prescribed by a professional practitioner of Chinese medicine they are effective, safe, and without side effects. In addition, they are usually much cheaper than modern Western pharmaceuticals.

And lastly, even though this is not a complete or word for word translation, we have chosen to retain the social and political comments of the Chinese original. Some of the statements regarding the benefits of socialism and modern science may appear quaint and dated. We debated deleting these as irrelevant to the needs and opinions of Western patients and practitioners but finally decided to keep them as a reminder that this book, like any book, is a product of a specific time and place and that, in assessing the relevance of any statement, we must always take into account the author's environment, beliefs, and unstated agenda.

Table of Contents

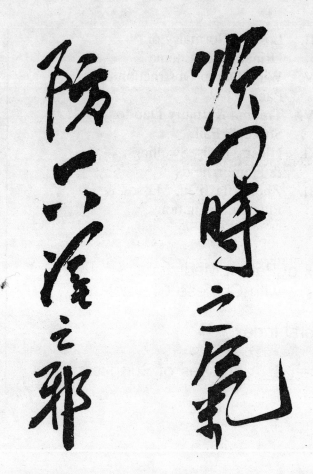

Follow the Qi of the four seasons,
Defend against the six wanton evils

1

Introduction

E veryone dreams of living longer and enjoying one's health in old age. Yet in ancient China where the political system was extremely rotten and science and medicine were not so advanced, people suffered from hunger and poverty. Life was difficult. No one dared dream of longevity and never mentioned a healthy, happy old age. Today socialism has brought the people better living conditions and provides a basic guarantee that older people should enjoy a better and healthier old age. On top of that, the development of modern science and improvements in everyday life and medical care all help make the dream of longevity come true.

How long can a human being live? Based on ancient medical records and scientific statistics on the age of the elderly in China and abroad, the answer is more than 100 years. This fact is also recorded in the *Nei Jing*, China's ancient medical classic which is more than 2,000 years old.

> In ancient times, those people who understood the *Dao* patterned their lives on yin and yang and lived in harmony through the arts of divination. They exercised temperance in eating and drinking. They regulated their hours of rising and retiring and were not disorderly and wild. By these means, the ancients kept their bodies united with their *shen* spirit so as to

completely fulfill their Heavenly decreed span measuring unto a natural hundred years before they passed away.

Further it was said: "In harmony with the *Dao*, they could live more than 100 years and remain active without becoming decrepit because their virtue was perfect and never imperiled."

"They could live more than 100 years and remain active" means that if a human being follow's nature's laws and has a well balanced lifestyle consisting of diet, work, exercise, and rest without unrealistic desires, they can enjoy a strong physical body, fulfilling mental health, and can live till 100. In Chinese the phrase "Heavenly decreed span or years" is regularly taken to mean 100 years. Human being should regularly be able to live to 100 years. Further, Chinese use the phrase "after 100 years" to describe the death of a person thus also implying that a person should live 100 years.

Likewise, according to comparative scientific studies of animal mortality, humans should live till 100. This has been deduced in three ways: First, most animals live 8-10 times their age at puberty. If human puberty comes at around 14 or 15, then humans should live to 110 or 115 years of age. Secondly, in most animals, maximum age equals 5-7 times an animal's growth period. Since the human growth period is from 20-25 years, then maximum age for humans should be 100-175 years old. And third, one can also count the number of cellular divisions to determine maximum lifespan. Human beings have around 50,000,000,000,000 cells which have divided over fifty times since the fetus. According to these calculations, human life should reach 110 years old. Some scientific researchers not only agree with the theory that humans should be able to live till 100 but also note that every species has their own particular life cycle which varies from a couple of seconds to thousands of years. For instance, rats have a 3 1/2 year life cycle, chickens a 30 year life cycle, and turtles have a 175 year life cycle.

The above considerations regarding human mortality are corroborated by the lives of numerous living elderly around the world. There are many people both in China and in other parts of the world who live past 100. Some areas are even known for their longevity. In China, there have been people who were 155 years old. In Burma, there have been people 168 years old. In Japan, 194 years old. In South America, 203 years old. In England, 209 years old. In Guangxi, a 90 something year old lady is still cooking, taking care of children, and enjoying her other jobs. An old French doctor continues his medical research at 103. In Columbia, a 132 year old man enjoys good health, singing and dancing full of vital energy. In Guangxi, there are more than 13 centenarians per 100,000 in the population. This fact proves that the percentage of centenarians is increasing.

However, there are lots of elderly people who die at 70 or 80 from disease and not from natural death. This happens in both in China and other countries. The elderly today are especially dying of heart disease, cancer, and respiratory diseases. These are the major causes of death in the elderly today. If we can treat these three categories of disease, the health and longevity of the elderly can be improved. Due to developments in science, medicine, and economic conditions, the general lifespan has gradually increased. This is especially so in countries were science and economics are both highly developed. China's average lifespan has also increased during the past 30 years. In Shanghai, China's most advanced city, everyone's life expectancy is 30 years more than in the past.

As the above clearly suggests, longer life most definitely can be achieved.

I. Signs of Health or Early Aging in the Elderly

In China, laypersons typically use the criteria of lack of blurred vision, lack of deafness, and lack of bowed back and weak knees to describe good health in the elderly. However, according to Traditional Chinese Medicine, a healthy elderly person is said to possess both *xing* and *shen*. What do *xing* and *shen* mean in this context? To explain this, we need to look at human physiology from the Chinese medical point of view.

Chinese medicine classifies the liver, heart, spleen, lungs, and kidneys as the five *zang* organs. Although each of these have their own individual physiological functions, these five organs are strongly tied to each other forming a totally undivided organism supporting the various functions of human life. Each organ has its own paired *fu* or bowel and its associated channel or meridian. In addition, skin, bone, sinews, and marrow are categorized according to their organ correspondences. The essential materials that fuel the body's normal physiologic activities are called *jing* or essence. Whereas, these normal physiological activities themselves are the manifestation of qi. The phrase "possessing both *xing* and *shen*" refers to a person's normal, everyday functioning. *Xing* means the physical body and *shen* refers to a person's spirit. If the physical body is strong, a person's life will be vivacious and full of energy, i.e. spirited. This means they possess both *xing* and *shen*. Whether a person possesses both *xing* and *shen* totally depends on the amount of their *jing* and qi. And this, in turn, is dependent upon the normal functioning of their *zang* and *fu*.

Jing is also called *yin jing*, in which case it includes *jing*, blood, and *jin ye*. *Jing* is the root of the body and blood is its support. Therefore, *jing* and blood are the material basis for the functioning of the all the organs in their entirety. When *jing* and blood are abundant, people enjoy better health. "When blood is abundant, the body (*xing*) is strong."

Qi means *yang qi*. This unequivocally refers to functional activity. Fullness (*shi*) or emptiness (*xu*) of the five *zang* are directly equated to the fullness or emptiness of their qi. For example, fullness or emptiness of the heart, kidneys, spleen, liver, or lung qi equals excess or deficiency of their functioning. Qi can also be categorized as *yuan qi, zhong qi, zong qi, ying qi,* and *wei qi*. *Yang qi* and *yin qi* are interdependent. *Yin qi* supports the existence of *yang qi* and *vice versa*. When *jing* is sufficient, qi is fulfilled. When qi is full, *shen* is strong. Therefore, we can say that *shen* is strongly related to *yang qi*. This also means that *shen* is the outer manifestation of qi. When qi and blood are harmonious, people are free from disease.

Jing, qi and *shen* are the general basis for human physical functioning. However, the five *zang* each have their own individual functions and their associated bowels and tissues.

The liver with its associated *fu* bowel, the gallbladder, controls the emotions and stores blood. It also governs the sinews, the nails, and the eyes. When liver blood is rich, both the sinews and the nails receive their nutrition via the blood. This manifests as flexible joints. But when one becomes old and weak, liver blood becomes insufficient and, therefore, the sinews lack their proper nutrition and thus the joints become inflexible. Motion becomes slower and muscles spasm more easily. In addition, the nails become thinner, whiter, and more brittle. "Liver qi goes to the eyes; when the liver is harmonious, the eyes can distinguish the five colors." It is liver blood which enables sight. When people get old and they still enjoy good eyesight, it means that liver blood is sufficient. Otherwise, if liver blood is empty, people complain of decreasing eyesight, blurring of vision, and/or dry eyes.

The heart with its associated bowel, the small intestine, controls the blood vessels and mental activity. It is said, "(The heart) controls the blood and the *shen ming* or the clarity of mental activity." It also guides the physiological activities and strength of the entire body. "The heart is the great ruler of the five *zang* and six *fu*." The functioning of the heart is closely connected with the tongue, the facial color, and perspiration. In Chinese medicine we say, "The tongue is the orifice of the heart" and that, "Sweat is the fluid of the heart." If the heart enjoys normal functioning as one ages, the pulse is even and strong and the circulation is free. This means that heart qi is strong and blood is rich. If the heart qi is weak and yin is empty, it will manifest as a weak or irregular pulse with a pale face, palpitations, and restlessness. Stagnation of heart blood manifests as a purple colored facial complexion and pain in the chest which radiates to the back. When blood and yin cannot nourish the heart, "the *shen* becomes homeless." This causes palpitations, insomnia, and disturbed dreams.

The spleen's associated bowel is the stomach. The stomach receives the food and initiates digestion. It "contains and receives" and "rotten and ripens". The spleen plays a role in further digestion and absorption and in the transportation of the food. Because of the relationship of the spleen to the transportation and transformation of food and liquids in the body, we say that the spleen is the root of acquisition and the source of growth and transformation. Good nutrition produces strong, well-built muscles and solid and strong limbs. It is said,

6

"The spleen rules the muscles and flesh," "(The spleen) rules the four extremities", and that its "orifice is the lips." When the spleen is strong, blood is sufficient since the spleen is the source of blood production. When old people enjoy a good appetite and digestion, this shows that the function of the spleen is good. When spleen function is weak, they suffer from poor digestion and abdominal bloating, loss of muscle tone, and weakness of the limbs. Their face may become either yellow or puffy.

The lungs' associated bowel is the large intestine. The lungs control breathing. Inhaled air combines in the lungs with the essence of water and grains (i.e., food and water) extracted by the spleen to become *zong* or ancestral or chest qi. *Zong qi* enables the circulation of qi and blood to nourish the entire body and maintain good functioning of the various organs. It is said, "The lungs govern depurative downbearing, they maintain the regular flow of the water passageways, and they transport (fluids) downward to the bladder." The lungs are also related to the hair and skin and the sense of smell. It is said, "The lungs govern the skin and hair and open into the nose." If an elderly person has weak lungs, they may suffer from cough, asthma, and dry skin and body hair. They will tend to catch cold easily and there may be shortness of breath. A person with strong lungs will not have these symptoms.

The kidneys with their associated bowel, the bladder, store the *jing* of the *zang* and *fu*. They have a strong relationship to growth, maturation, and reproduction in the human being. They control the bones, marrow, and teeth. Likewise, hearing and the growth of head hair are also dependent on kidney function. Therefore in Chinese medicine we say, "The orifice of the kidneys are the ears and the glory of the kidneys manifests in the hair." The excretion of liquids requires kidney qi to speed it on its way in addition to the qi of the lungs and spleen. Whereas, the bladder only stores the urine, kidney qi controls the opening and closing of the bladder. When old people suffer from deafness, dizziness, loose teeth, falling hair, weak knees and difficulty walking, sore lower back, impotence, and polyuria, these are all symptoms of emptiness of kidney qi.

From the above discussion it is clear that each of the five *zang* have their own functions and characteristics, but, in sum, we can use the saying, "possessing both *xing* and *shen*" to describe a healthy older person.

II. The Causes of Premature Aging And Geriatric Disease

Birth, growth, old age, and death are the natural order which no life can resist. Without birth there can be no death and *vice versa*. Life and death together form a circle which rolls on forever. Human beings are not outside this natural condition.

All animals have their own life cycle of growth and decline. What is the rule for human beings? The *Nei Jing* says:

> When one is 10 years old, one's five *zang* begin to grow, one's qi and blood circulate, and all the qi goes downward so one becomes better at walking. When 20 years old, qi and blood become strong, the muscles are firm, and so one becomes good at fast walking. When 30 years old, the five *zang* are all solidly built and the muscles are strongly formed. One's blood vessels are full so on is good at running. When 40 years old, the five *zang* and six *fu* along with

the twelve channels are over their peak and are starting to decline. The hair starts to turn grey and one is good at sitting. When one is 50 years old, liver qi starts to decline and gallbladder juice begins to decrease. Therefore the eyesight begins to blur. When 60 years old, heart qi begins to weaken, qi and blood are both becoming slack, and so one tends to sleep more. When 70 years old, spleen qi is weak and the skin is dry. When 80 years old, lung qi declines and the po leaves the body, so one's speech is not clear. When 90 years old, kidney qi is burning out and the four zang and channels and vessels are empty. When 100 years old, the five zang are empty, the shen and qi are gone, and thus one is ready to depart.

Although this description may seem overly mechanical, yet it does reflect the overall life cycle of a human being's birth, growth, and death.

Human beings cannot change the order of birth and death. However, humans can actively improve upon this cycle and delay premature aging. Conversely, peoples' wrong doing can negatively affect this scenario. Our ancestors paid great attention to their lifestyle and this had a major impact on prolonging their lifespan and preventing premature debility and death. They also remind us of the harmful effects of not keeping a good lifestyle. As the *Nei Jing* says:

Nowadays people are not like this. They use wine as a beverage and they adopt recklessness and unusual behavior. They enter the chamber in an intoxicated condition (i.e., have sex while drunk) and their passions exhaust their vital forces. Their cravings dissipate their true essence and they do not know how to find contentment within themselves. They are not skilled in the control of their Spirits and they devote all their attention to the amusement of their minds. Thus they cut themselves off from the joys of long life. Their rising and retiring is without regularity. For these reasons they reach only one half of their 100 years and they degenerate.

The above statements are both correct and practical and are supported by modern medical theory and clinical experience. When a person does not know how to restrict their own action and thus indulges in a lifestyle of overeating, overdrinking, and too much sex, one will never have a healthy longevity. One cannot but have a short life.

Chinese medicine divides the causes of disease into 1) the six evil qi, 2) the seven passions, and 3) diet and stress.

Wind, cold, summer heat, dampness, dryness, and heat are called the six qi (*liu qi*) when they are normal. The six qi describe the fluctuations and progressions in the weather and climate throughout the year. This is according to natural law. The human body needs these changes and automatically adjusts to and can cope with them during our everyday life. Therefore, the six qi are not harmful to the body. But, if the six qi are excess or deficient, this is not natural. If one of them comes at the wrong time or lingers too long, if it comes too abundantly, if it gets too hot when it is not supposed to or too cold when winter has not yet arrived, all these abnormalities can directly influence our daily physical routine and cause illness to occur. In such cases, the six qi become the six evils (*liu xie*). In everyday life, it is easier for us to catch a cold when the weather suddenly changes too hot or too cold. When we suddenly move from one climate to another, if we cannot cope with the new environment, we will be affected by the six evil qi and become sick. Sometimes, even when the six qi are normal, we may still catch disease if we do not pay attention to wearing proper clothes or when our immune system is depressed.

As people age, one's *jing qi* becomes deficient and weak, one's five *zang* wane, and their *zheng* or righteous qi becomes insufficient. Thus the six evil qi can easily invade the bodies of the elderly and cause disease. Therefore it is common to see old people suffering from recurrent asthma or cough as winter approaches or sudden collapse and death during the extreme heat of summer or cold of winter. In short, older people are more easily attacked by the six evil qi.

The emotional factors which cause disease are joy, anger, brooding, sadness, and fear or fright. Under normal circumstances, these emotions are the appropriate reflection internally of stimuli from the outside world. Crying, laughing, and being happy are feelings normal to the human body. When they are not out of control, they do not adversely affect the *zang fu* and no disease ensues. But, when they are out of control, excessive anger can injure the liver, excessive joy can injure the heart, excessive brooding can injure the spleen, excessive sadness can injure the lungs, and excessive fright can injure the kidneys. Anger arouses the ascent of qi. Joy induces sluggishness of the qi. Excessive sorrow dissipates the qi. Fear causes the descent of the qi. Fright causes disturbance of the qi. And worry causes stagnation of qi.

Although it may at first sound peculiar that emotions may injure or kill a person, in fact, this happens every day. Chinese people are wont to say, "I laughed myself to death," or "I'm so sad I'm dying." These are vivid examples of the reality of this proposition. We have heard of elderly people dying due to sudden joy causing an unstoppable fit of laughter. We have also heard of some elderly persons dying of heart attack caused by a sudden increase in blood pressure in turn due to getting angry. Overthinking can harm the functions of the heart and spleen and liver and spleen which will then manifest such symptoms as anxiety, insomnia, tenderness of the hypochondrium, dizziness, belching, bloating, and decreased appetite. These days, authorities from various countries agree that there is a relationship between cancer and emotional stress or imbalance. When a person suffers from longterm, extreme depression, anger, sadness, or worry, they can develop cancer. Because of their emptiness of *jing* and qi, the elderly are all the more easily injured by uncontrollable emotions.

Irregular diet includes both overeating and undereating. It also includes eating too much raw, cold food, hot foods, and oily, greasy, or spicy foods. All of these can cause disharmony of the *zang fu*. Such dietary irregularities first attack the stomach/spleen. This then escalates from mild digestive disturbance to severe disease due to spleen dysfunction failing to perform its functions of transportation and transformation. Poor digestion is a common problem amongst the elderly. Therefore, they need to be more careful than others with their diet. Unfortunately, some people simply ignore their health and lose control during the holiday seasons. They overeat and overdrink at family reunions which cause them immediate woe.

In Chinese medicine, stress means overtaxing the body or overconsuming our body's energy. This includes too much sex. Too much sex causes more harm than most people think. It is a major cause of kidney emptiness. Too much sex exhausts kidney *jing* and leads to emptiness of both kidney yin and yang.

This manifests as loss of teeth, low back weakness and pain, difficulty walking, dizziness, and premature ejaculation or impotence. Too much sex, *fang lao* in Chinese or literally bedroom taxation, is very harmful to the elderly. Therefore, they should not ignore this.

III. The *Dao* of Increasing Longevity And Conserving One's Life

To reiterate the above, in conjunction with tonifying their *zheng* or righteous qi, we know that the elderly need to pay particular attention to the following guidelines in maintaining their health and thus securing longevity.

A.   *Qi Ju You Chang,*
       Lao Yi Shi Du

     A constant and regular lifestyle,
     Suitable amounts of work and rest

What were our ancestors' secrets for attaining longevity? One answer is, "A constant and regular lifestyle (and) suitable amounts of work and rest." This saying implies that there should be a certain regimen to our life which includes reasonable amounts of working time, rest, exercise, and sleep.

According to the *Nei Jing*, one should go to bed late, rise early, and take a walk in the spring. During the summer, one should go to bed late and rise early being sure to spend a good bit of time out of doors. In the fall, one should go to bed early and get up early, and during the winter one should go to bed early and get up late. Whether or not this theory is scientific requires further investigation. Nonetheless, during the spring

13

and summer when all things are growing and the weather is warm and nice, it is certainly healthy for us to take a walk in the sun and inhale the fresh air outdoors. During the autumn, the sky is high, the air is clear, and the weather is comfortable. Daylight grows less and the night is longer each day. So it is also healthy for the body to take a walk outdoors and inhale the fresh air. Because it is so cold during winter, we should avoid chilly mornings and wait for the warm sunshine in order to prevent attacks of cold evils. According to foreign studies, early risers indeed do enjoy longer life. In Japan, all the elderly of unusually advanced years get up from 4-6 AM. That is the time when all the birds wake. Chinese medicine recommends that everyone get up early during the spring, summer, and fall and wake up late during the winter. This follows the same belief as the long-lived in Japan.

During one's older year, the *jing qi* is generally weakened and depleted. *Zang fu* function is not as energetic and strong as in youth. It is therefore of utmost importance to avoid hard labor and to pay attention to resting and fostering the needs of the body. To get sufficient sleep is also very important. Good sleep helps our *shen* reside within the body unperturbed by the outside world. Thus it is a well accepted theory among people that the key to longevity is the ability to eat and sleep well. In everyday life, we often encounter people in poor health due to insomnia and they are invariably fatigued and their memory is poor. When this happens in the elderly, it speeds up the aging process. Thus a good balance between physical labor and mental activity is recommended. It is a proven fact that enjoying pleasant music can increase both one's physical and emotional strength. Taking a walk after meals improves the digestion. Further, gardening, enjoying keeping fish in the house, and playing various Chinese games are all species of active rest which each individual can chose according to their individual preference.

14

Rest and exercise should complement one another. Rest alone with little if any physical exertion tends to be harmful to the body. Chinese medicine regards longterm sitting as harmful to our muscles and longterm lying down as harmful to our qi. It can therefore be concluded that good diet and rest alone without physical exercise, in fact, overburdens the body and thus weakens the entire system. The *Nei Jing* calls this, "bodily exhaustion not due to fatigue". As Sun Si-miao of the Tang Dynasty said, "In order for the body to feel comfortable and healthy, we need suitable amounts of labor." Modern medicine has proven that decrease in muscle tone due to lack of exercise also results in decreases in the tone and functioning of the nervous, circulatory, and digestive systems and accelerates the aging process. In addition, lack of exercise and too much stress are also causes of heart and cerebral ischemic disease. Therefore, older persons are recommended to choose suitable, individualized exercise to retard aging. This includes *Qi Gong, Tai Ji Quan*, walking, etc. Each individual can chose different activities. Whatever the exercise, one should feel well and refreshed after each session. One should also be aware that, "Lifting things which are beyond our strength will cause more harm to the body."

B.   *Shun Si Shi Zhi Qi,*
      Fang Liu Yin Zhi Xie

      Follow the qi of the four seasons,
      Defend against the six wanton evils

According to Traditional Chinese Medicine, in order to conserve one's life, people should live in consonance with the changes of the four seasons and yin and yang qi. Our bodies and our lives should be in harmony with nature and thus remain in a well balanced state. As it is said, "Harmonize with yin and yang and balance with the four seasons." It is also said, "Going against causes harm, while following along results in health; this is the *Dao*." *Dao* means rules and laws or the rules of conserving one's life. The *Nei Jing* mentions again and again the harmful effects the changing of the four seasons can have on the human body. It is said, "One should avoid all emptiness and evils and especially evil wind," and, "The sage avoids emptiness and evils as he would attack by stones." These sayings remind us to avoid the evil qi of the four seasons and to avoid attack by external evils. Dr. Yi Shi of the Ming Dynasty advised weakened persons to be especially aware of the following: to defend against wind in spring; to defend against summer heat in summer; to defend against dampness in late summer; to defend against dryness in fall; to defend against cold in winter; and to also defend against warmness when the season is not supposed to be warm such as in the winter. Following such advice by the ancients is important for maintaining health and should not be neglected by the elderly.

The ability of the elderly to adjust to changeable weather is weak. Therefore, they need to pay special attention to these instructions and also to the way they dress and eat. One should not let external evils attack through the skin and hair, i.e., the surface, nor should one allow them to attack through the mouth and nose. In sum, "One must pay attention to adjust when the seasons are changeable."

C.   *Yi Le Guan Kai Lang,*
•   *Fang Qing Xu Ju Bian*

       Be happy with a light, open view;
       Guard against being seized by sudden
           changes in emotion

As mentioned above, when the so-called seven passions or emotions are grossly excessive, they can injure a person. Dr. Sun Xi-miao of the Qing Dynasty said:

> To live long, people should take care not to worry too much, not to get too angry, not to get too sad, not to get frightened, not to do too much, talk too much, or laugh too much. One should not have too many desires nor face numerous upsetting conditions. All these are harmful to the health.

He also said:

> One who knows how to conserve one's life is one who thinks less, worries less, has less desire, is less active, talks less, is less upset, has less joy, has less anger, and does less wrong. These twelve lesses are the key to conserving one's life.

An individual is but a small part of society and has strong ties to society. Therefore the "twelve lesses" are difficult to follow and not even entirely correct. We do need to worry for our society and our country and to make our contribution to society. Therefore, some of the twelve lesses are not totally right. However, from the point of view of conserving one's life, the emphasis should be on the word less which means avoiding _extreme_ emotional ups and downs. Studies show that talking increases the blood pressure in patients with hypertension. We need to have a broad, open mind with a happy mood and avoid all _unnecessary_ worries and stress. One should not run after fame or money. Therefore, the saying, "A broad mind, a healthy body," proves to be very true. Li Ma-kang, a centenarian from Beijing has said that the secret of his longevity was to 1) never worry and 2) not to overeat.

The emotional well-being of the elderly depends both upon the individual and upon society and one's family. Our excellent socialism gives all older persons a very happy life. There is the Society for Respecting the Elderly which provides a place for all old people who are alone. We also recommend the good habit of respecting and loving the aged. And we strongly criticize any maltreatment or disrespect of older people. Rather we should make them feel comfortable no matter where they are, whether at home or in public.

D.   *Yin Shi You Jie*
      Ji Bao Yin Bao Shi

      Be abstinent in food and drink;
      Refrain from eating and drinking till you bulge

Diet is the key to bodily health. There can be no healthy body without a healthy diet. Overeating and inappropriate foods harm the body. As our ancestors said,

      Care of the body depends upon diet. Being
      drunk yet longing to drink more, being full yet
      craving to eat more are major impediments on
      the path to *yang shéng* or lengthening life.

It is important for the elderly to have a well regulated diet. Overeating and overdrinking are harmful. In maintaining a better balanced diet and hence a healthy body, it is wise to eat more vegetables and bean products such as tofu. Vegetables stimulate the secretive functions of various glands within the body. Vegetables are easily digested and assimilated by the body. They can increase intestinal peristalsis and improve

18

/bowel movements. They can detoxify. They also prevent obesity, diabetes, heart disease, and other disorders. As one ages, the functioning of the *zang* and *fu* becomes debilitated. Therefore it is important for the elderly not to overeat. Overeating high cholesterol and high calorie food is generally the cause of cancer, arteriosclerosis, coronary heart disease, hypertension, and premature aging. The *Nei Jing* states that *xiao ke* or diabetes (literally thirsting & wasting) is caused by "all fat, greasy, oily foods". One should not be prejudiced in favor of a particular food. In Guangxi, one centenarian eats mainly vegetables, the five grains, and little animal products. His main foods are cereal and bean products like tofu and vegetables cooked in sesame oil. This kind of food provides less calories but more of the nutrients the body needs. It maintains good stomach/spleen function for digestion and assimilation and guarantees strong transportation and transformation, hence a healthy body.

It is advisable for the elderly not to overeat in order for them to keep their *fu* bowels free flowing. The *fu* bowels need to be free flowing at all times. Overeating impedes their function and causes food stagnation. This results in intestinal bloating and distention, indigestion, and loss of appetite. This can further affect the function of other organs and will eventually affect the functioning of the entire body. One should eat less food and food which is easy to digest, especially for dinner. Chinese believe that everyone should have a full breakfast, a good lunch, and a light dinner.

In treating patients with Chinese medicine, vinegar and alcohol are often used. Vinegar penetrates the liver channel and assists the liver in its dispersion of the qi. It also indirectly assists digestion and benefits the stomach/spleen. This is the reason why many dispersing herbs are prepared with vinegar.

Rice wine, on the other hand, helps promote the circulation of qi and blood within the channels and connecting vessels as well as strengthens the muscles and sinews. This does not mean patients should mistakenly overconsume these two products based on the above medical concepts. For instance, if rice wine is overconsumed, its longterm consequences can include high blood pressure, arteriosclerosis, and hepatitis. These products should only be used medicinally to assist in achieving health.

Drinking tea in suitable amounts is also good for the body. As an herbal medicinal, drinking tea can "make people strong and comfortable feeling"; "it disinhibits urination, clears hot phlegm, eliminates thirst, and can also improve digestion." According to an ancient, Tang Dynasty classic, it can treat diarrhea and alcohol toxins. Modern studies show that tea leaves have, besides vitamins A, B_2, and C, caffeine. Caffeine can excite the nervous system, activate the mind, and help one recover from fatigue. It can also excite the heart, enlarge the coronary artery, and increase the blood supply to the heart. It can especially disinhibit urination and increase the secretion of stomach juices to help digestion. It can relax the smooth muscles in the treatment of bronchial asthma and cholecystitis. It kills germs and stops bleeding. When tea is combined with other toxic foods, it can slow down the absorption of those toxins. Therefore, it can detoxify. Drinking tea can increase the excretion of alcohol which thus reduces toxicity in the liver. It can also decrease fat deposits, prevents obesity, and also dispels phlegm. It is good for treating diabetes.

Drinking tea in suitable amounts is good for the elderly. Yet overdrinking tea can be harmful in the long run. It is especially ill advised to drink strong tea if one has high blood pressure, insomnia, or stomach ulcers. The best time to drink tea is after meals and one should not oversoak the tea leaves as this can cause constipation.

2

Chinese Patent Medicines Appropriate for Supplementing & Boosting Emptiness & Weakness in Those With Emptiness, Weakness, & Decline of the Body

W hat is generally referred to as physical or constitutional emptiness feebleness (*xu ruo*) is also called, in Chinese medicine, emptiness, feebleness, deficit, and decrease of the body (*xing ti xu ruo kui sun*), emptiness & decrease (*xu sun*, which implies a species of damage due to emptiness), emptiness taxation (*xu lao*), major deficit of source qi (*yuan qi da kui*), and decrease & injury of the five *zang* (*wu zang sun shang*). The Sui Dynasty *Chao Shi Bing Yuan* (*Chao's Source of Disease*) categorizes and elucidates *xu lao* or emptiness taxation by saying, "emptiness taxation is due to the five taxations (*wu lao*), the six extremes (*liu ji*), or the seven injuries (*qi shang*)."

The five taxations each correspond to an taxation of one of the five *zang*. When the heart is overtaxed, this harms the blood. When the liver is overtaxed, this harms the *shen*. When the spleen is overtaxed, this harms the appetite and digestion. When the lungs are overtaxed, this harms the circulation of qi. When the kidneys are overtaxed, this harms the *jing*.

The six extremes describe diseases caused by six types of extreme emptiness. So-called blood extreme (*xue ji*) results in hair loss and poor memory. Sinew extreme (*jin ji*) manifests as spasms of the muscles and tendons. Flesh extreme (*rou ji*) manifests as pallor and emaciation. Qi extreme (*qi ji*) manifests as shortness of breath and asthmatic conditions. Bone extreme (*gu ji*) manifests as loss of teeth and *wei zheng* or flaccidity syndrome of the legs. And essence extreme (*jing ji*) manifests as weakening of the eyesight and deafness.

The seven injuries or *qi shang* are described as follows: Overeating injures the spleen. Heavy lifting or excessive sitting on wet ground over a long period inures the kidneys. Cold drinks injure the lungs. Worry injures the heart. Wind, rain, cold, and heat injure the *xing* or body. Extreme anger injures the liver. And fright injures the *zhi* or will.

Emptiness aside from the above may be induced by other factors, a number of which are described as follows:

1. A congenitally weak constitution coupled with lack of proper nutrition during growth as well as loss of *jing* and blood may all contribute to emptiness of the *yuan qi*.

2. Chronic, consumptive diseases weaken the *zheng qi*. While overeating greasy, spicy food, overdrinking of alcohol, and sexual taxation bring harm to the stomach/spleen and weaken the *jing qi*.

3. Maladaptation to seasonal and environmental changes can result in the body's abuse by the six evil qi. Prolonged or recurrent conditions harm both the qi and the blood.

4. Overtaxation by the seven passions results in imbalance among the *zang* and *fu*. Over a period of time, this will harm

22

the *zheng qi*.

Premature aging and weakening of the body is prompted by imbalance in living one's daily life and this is especially so for the elderly.

Xu sun typically presents as such symptoms as whole body weakness, shortness of breath, spontaneous perspiration, palpitations, fatigue, facial pallor, weight loss, loss of appetite, poor digestion, dizziness, tinnitus, deafness, loss of teeth and hair, weakness and soreness of the low back and knees, difficulty walking, and urinary and fecal incontinence. Of course this is just a general list of signs and symptoms and not all of these will necessarily present simultaneously.

There are other conditions, such as emptiness of qi and blood, a tendency to yang qi emptiness, and exhaustion of blood and *jing*, which may be associated with *xu sun*. Thus in treating various species of *xu sun*, various different patent medicines are used. The reader should be aware that supplementing medications will only benefit a patient who is diagnosed as empty. If used in fullness patterns (*shi zheng*), they will increase this fullness and therefore cause additional harm leading to a further imbalance of yin and yang. Caution must be taken when warm, dry tonics such as Radix Panacis Ginseng and Cornu Cervi Parvum are used since their warm nature may damage yin and create full fire.

I. Qi & Blood Supplementation

Qi is united with the blood. Together they are the fountainhead and spring of the body's biological activities and strength. The condition of the body, whether full or empty, is

23

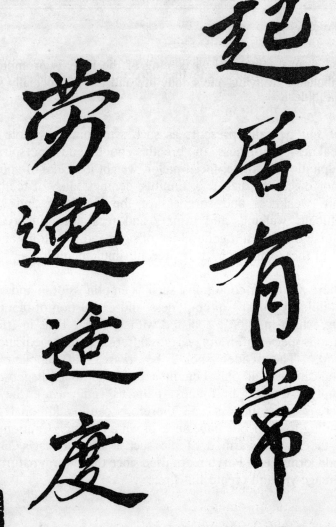

A constant and regular lifestyle,
Suitable amounts of work and rest

closely related to the qi and blood. Qi describes the quality of the functioning of the entire body. When righteous qi is sufficient, body function is active and strong. When righteous qi declines or wanes, body function becomes sluggish and weak. The qi of the body may be divided into *yuan qi, zong qi, ying qi, wei qi*, and the qi of the five *zang*.

Yuan qi or *yuan yang* is the prenatal qi inherited from the parents. It is stored within the kidney *jing* and is transformed and created from the kidney essence. It moves throughou the whole body and it catalyzes the body's functions. It promotes the strength of the five *zang* and six *fu* and is the source of activity and strength of the entire human body. The strength and activity of one's life force is dependent upon this original strength. Therefore, the *yuan qi* is correctly called the root qi of the human body. The strength or weakness of *yuan qi* depends upon our inheritance from our parents and acquired qi derived from nutrition during the process of growth.

The fact that *yuan qi* is technically described as prenatal does not imply that it cannot be either strengthened or weakened postnatally. Due to taxation of kidney *jing* in the elderly, *yuan qi* is gradually weakened. Thus the elderly, once they become empty, need to be administered appropriate supplementary medicinals to maintain strong, healthy *yuan qi*.

Zong or chest qi is a combination of both nutrients absorbed by the stomach/spleen and air inhaled into the chest. It resides in the chest and promotes the activity of the heart and lungs. It is the acquired root which governs the quality of our bodily functioning. In addition, it can resupply emptiness of *yuan qi*. Emptiness of chest qi results in shortness of breath, a weakened heart and thus decreased heart rate, and a weakened voice.

Wei qi is our protective qi. It warms the skin, protects the

25

superficial level of the body, maintains body temperature, and resists invasion by external evil qi. Its state or condition is directly related to the *yuan qi* and chest qi. It is believed that *wei qi* is derived from *yuan qi* and chest qi. Emptiness of *wei qi* leaves the body unguarded against abuse and invasion by evil qi.

The five *zang qi* refer to lung qi, heart qi, middle qi, etc. A person suffering from *qi xu* or qi emptiness (which includes chest qi emptiness) exhibits signs of lethargy, a low, weak voice, easy perspiration, dizziness, palpitations, tinnitus, fatigue, lack of appetite, abdominal bloating, and a weak pulse.

Blood is transformed by qi from the nutrients acquired from food. Strong, healthy stomach/spleen function transports and transforms food; thus qi generates and transforms the blood. It is therefore reasonable to assume that by supplementing spleen qi and promoting spleen function, qi will generate and transform blood. This is the basis of the concept, "When nourishing the blood, also supplement the qi."

Kidney *jing* can also be transformed into blood and *vice versa*. This is the reason why *jing* and blood can transform into one another and mutually promote each other's growth. Hence, whenever supplementing the kidneys, one should also supplement the liver. Abundance of kidney *jing* enriches the blood and its emptiness results in emptiness of the blood.

The function of the blood or *xue* is to nourish the body. The ability to see, walk, hold things in our hands, and have a full head of hair, well nourished muscles and tendons, and smooth, lustrous skin are all based on the blood's function of nourishing. Therefore we can say that blood is the material basis of our life force.

Spleen and stomach emptiness results in inhibition of transportation and transformation. The food consumed is not then transformed adequately into blood. By the same token, when blood is empty due to longterm weakness, there will be such symptoms as pallor, brittle nails, dizziness, palpitations, fatigue, spasm of the muscles and tendons, and numbness.

Thus qi and blood emptiness manifest as emptiness and Decline of the entire body and therefore patent medicines appropriate for the supplementation of this type of emptiness should be able to benefit and supplement *yuan qi*, spleen qi, and lung qi. Such medicinals promote the body's activity and strength, enhance its metabolism, nourish the blood, and benefit the body as a whole.

```
Legend:
★      =       Available from   Mayway
♦      =       "      "         Nuherbs
●      =       "   as a powdered extract
```

Du Shen Tang ★♦
Ren Shen Jing ★♦
Ren Shen Tang ★♦

Ingredients: These three patent medicines are all composed of the single medicinal ingredient Radix Panacis Ginseng. *Du Shen Tang* is a soup or decoction made from Ginseng; *Ren Shen Jing* is a liquid extract; and *Ren Shen Tang* is a sugar crystal/ginseng preparation.

Indications: These medicines are all used for *xu sun* or

27

emptiness weakness with loss of appetite, fatigue, nausea, vomiting, diarrhea, asthma, cough, palpitations, forgetfulness, headache and dizziness, impotence, polyuria, diabetes, stroke, pallor, cold limbs, profuse perspiration, and a weak pulse.

Shen Qi Jing ♦

Ingredients: This is an extract made from Radix Panacis Ginseng and Radix Astragali Seu Hedysari.

Indications: Weakness, loss of appetite, fatigue, and insomnia in conjunction with other qi, blood, and body fluids emptiness signs and symptoms

Shen Qi Da Bu Wan ★

Ingredients: These pills are composed of Radix Codonopsis Pilosulae and Radix Astragali Seu Hedysari.

Indications: Weakness, diabetes, profuse, daytime perspiration, fatigue, and loss of appetite. Naeser indicates it for emptiness of qi due to long time illness, blood loss, or postpartum weakness. It supplements the qi and strengthens the spleen. Zhu adds that this medication treats emptiness of middle qi due to longterm illness and also that it treats emaciation.

Bei Qi Jing ★♦
Zeng Bei Qi Pian ★♦
Bei Qi Jing ★♦

Ingredients: *Bei Qi Jing* is an extract composed of Radix Astragali Seu Hedysari and honey; *Zheng Bei Qi Pian* are tablets composed of astragalus; and *Bei Qi Jing* are crystals made from astragalus.

Indications: Emptiness of both qi and blood, surface emptiness with perspiration, weakness of the four limbs, loss of energy, or emptiness and weakness of the stomach/spleen during convalescence from a chronic disease. Fratkin says that this patent medicine supplements spleen qi, *wei qi*, and blood. Besides helping recovery from chronic illness and childbirth, he also suggests it boosts immunity.

Shuang Bao Su Kou Fu Ye ★

Ingredients: This liquid is composed of Royal Jelly and Radix Panacis Ginseng.

Indications: Heart disease, hepatitis, anemia, premature, rheumatoid arthritis, stomach ulcers, neuralgia, balding, and constitutional emptiness after disease. Naeser says this medicine strengthens the qi, nourishes the liver, and supplements the spleen and that it is used to treat general weakness. Zhu refers to this medication as simply *Shuang Bao Su* .

Bei Jing Feng Wang Jing ★♦
Bei Jing Ling Zhi Feng Wang Jing ★♦
Bei Jing Feng Ru Jing Pian ★♦

Ingredients: *Bei Jjing Feng Wang Jjing* is a liquid extract composed of Royal Jelly, Radix Panacis Ginseng, Radix Codonopsis Pilosulae, Fructus Lycii Chinensis, Fructus Schizandrae Chinensis, and other undisclosed ingredients. *Bei Jing Ling Zhi Feng Wang Jing* is a liquid extract composed of Royal Jelly, Fructificatio Ganodermae Lucidi, Radix Polygoni Multiflori, Fructus Psoraleae Corylifoliae, Herba Epimedii, vitamins, etc. *Bei Jing Feng Ru Jing Pian* are tablets composed of Royal Jelly, Radix Panacis Ginseng, vitamin C, vitamin B_1, and vitamin B_2.

Indications: *Bei Jing Feng Wang Jing* is for lack of appetite, neurasthenia, anemia, stomach ulcers, premature aging, hepatitis, arthritis, and vasculitis. *Bei Jing Ling Zhi Feng Wang Jing* is for post disease constitutional emptiness, loss of appetite, neurasthenia, hepatitis, rheumatoid arthritis, anemia, stomach ulcers, etc. And *Bei Jing Feng Ru Jing Pian* is for premature aging, loss of appetite, rheumatoid arthritis, vasculitis, wind dampness, anemia, etc.

Naeser gives several additional liquid extract, qi and blood supplementing medicinals. These are *Ling Zhi Feng Wang Jiang* and *Ren Shen Feng Wang Jiang*. *Ling Zhi Feng Wang Jiang* is composed of Fructificatio Ganodermae Lucidi, Royal Jelly, Radix Codonopsis Pilosulae, and Fructus Lycii Chinensis. Naeser says this medication supplements and nourished qi and blood and is used to treat consumptive diseases as described above plus cancer. *Ren Shen Feng Wang Jiang* contains Radix Panacis Ginseng and Royal Jelly and Naeser says it is especially good for treating empty qi and yang.

Shen Qi Feng Wang Jiang ★♦

Ingredients: This liquid extract is composed Radix Panacis Ginseng, Radix Astragali Seu Hedysari, and Royal Jelly.

Indications: Emptiness of qi, taxation of blood, weakness, lack of appetite, anemia, and malnutrition

Feng Mi

Ingredients: This is simply honey.

Indications: Honey is a general supplementing medicinal which warms the middle burner and stops pain. It benefits empty cold stomach pain. It is good for heart disease, moistens the lungs, stops cough, and lubricates the intestines.

Ren Shen Feng Mi ★◆

Ingredients: Radix Panacis Ginseng and honey

Indications: Emptiness of both qi and blood, constitutional weakness, fatigue, cough, asthma, etc.

Ci Wu Jia Yang Shen Su ★◆
Wu Jia Shen Chong Ji ★◆
Wu Jia Shen Jing ★◆
Ci Wu Jia Pian ★◆

Ingredients: *Ci Wu Jia Yang Shen Su* is composed of Cortex Radicis Acanthopanacis plus A, B, C, D, and E vitamins. This herbal medicinal is similar to ginseng. It strengthens the body, strengthens the sinews and the bones, supplements the *zheng* or righteous qi, calms the spirit, tonifies the kidneys, strengthens the spleen, regulates the qi, and transforms phlegm.

Indications: These formulas, all of which are made from acanthopanax, are used for weakness, fatigue, lack of appetite, chronic bronchitis in the elderly, decreased libido, and insomnia due to chronic disease. According to Naeser, *Ci Wu Jia Pian* is indicated for the treatment of emptiness of qi with fatigue, dizziness, insomnia, and poor appetite and sexual dysfunction with spermatorrhea, impotence, and impaired sexual desire. Zhu specifies this medicine for emptiness of middle qi and that it is that emptiness which is responsible for the fatigue, dizziness, insomnia, and poor appetite. Zhu also recommends this medication for migraine headache due to emptiness of middle qi.

He Che Fen ★♦
Tai Pan Pian ★♦

Ingredients: *He Che Fen* is composed of Placenta Hominis. *Tai Pan Pian* is composed of Placenta Hominis and white sugar.

Indications: *He Che Fen* is for emptiness of both qi and blood, premature ejaculation, darkening of the facial complexion, and weakness of the bones and tendons. *Tai Pan Pian* is for asthma, night sweats, spermatorrhea, and decline of yang.

Ling Zhi Qiang Ti Pian ★

Ingredients: These tablets are composed of Radix Panacis Ginseng, Fructificatio Ganodermae Lucidi and other Chinese herbs which are unspecified.

Indications: Neurasthenia, palpitations, insomnia, loss of appetite, anemia, shortness of breath, hypertension, etc.

Yan Nian Yi Suo Jing ★

Ingredients: Not given. This medicine is based on a qing Dynasty formula called *Yan Nian Yi Shou Dan*, or *Postpone Aging & Benefit Longevity Elixir*.

Indications: Constitutional weakness due to aging

Shi Quan Da Bu Wan ★♦●

Ingredients: Radix Codonopsis Pilosulae, Radix Astragali Seu Hedysari, Cortex Cinnamomi, Radix Conquitae Rehmanniae, Rhizoma Atractylodis Macrocephalae, Radix Angelicae Sinensis, Radix Alba Paeoniae Lactiflorae, Radix Ligustici Wallichii, Sclerotium Poriae Cocoris, Radix Glycyrrhizae

Indications: Weakness caused by emptiness of both qi and blood, pallor, cough and asthma due to emptiness, fatigue, premature ejaculation, and weakness of the low back and knees. According to Naeser, *Shi Quan Da Bu Wan* supplements the qi and blood and is used to treat empty qi and general debility, uterine bleeding due to empty qi and blood, and spermatorrhea due to empty qi and blood. In addition, it can help treat chronic, subcutaneous skin ulcers, such as bedsores, which may be deep-rooted and long-standing. However, because Cortex Cinnamomi warms and consolidates kidney yang, Fratkin cautions that this medicine should be suspended if symptoms of heat develop.

Ren Shen Yang Rong Wan ★♦

Ingredients: Radix Panacis Ginseng, Rhizoma Atractylodis Macrocephalae, Sclerotium Poriae Cocoris, Radix Glycyrrhizae, Radix Angelicae Sinensis, Radix Conquita Rhemanniae, Radix Alba Paeoniae Lactiflorae, Radix Astragali Seu Hedysari, Cortex Cinnamomi, Pericarpium Citri Reticulatae, Radix Polygalae Tenuifoliae, Fructus Schizandrae Chinensis, Rhizoma Recens Zingiberis, Fructus Zizyphi Jujubae

Indications: Weakness due to emptiness of the heart and spleen, emptiness of both qi and blood, loss of appetite, loose stools, palpitations, and forgetfulness. Naeser says this medicine strengthens the qi and blood, calms the spirit, and improves the memory. It can be used to treat conditions related to either dual emptiness of the heart and spleen or empty yang of the spleen and kidneys.

Dang Gui Bu Xue Gao ★♦

Ingredients: This liquid medicine is composed of Radix Angelicae Sinensis, Radix Ligustici Wallichii, Radix Astragali

33

Seu Hedysari, Radix Glycyrrhizae, Radix Codonopsis Pilosulae, Radix Alba Paeoniae Lactiflorae, Gelatinum Asini, Sclerotium Poriae Cocoris, Radix Conquita Rehmanniae.

Indications: Weakness, dizziness, headache, anemia after disease, post partum emptiness of blood, etc. Naeser lists a seemingly identical Chinese patent medicine called *Dang Gui Yang Xue Gao* with the same ingredients. She gives the indications of it as empty blood symptoms, dizziness, palpitations, poor memory, fatigue, anemia, and gynecological disorders, such as scanty periods, amenorrhea, and post partum weakness due to blood loss.

Quan Lu Wan ★

Ingredients: This pill is composed of Caro Cervi, Cornu Parvum Cervi, Penis Et Testis Cervi, Renal Cervi, Gelatinum Cornu Cervi, Radix Panacis Ginseng, Rhizoma Atractylodis Macrocephalae, Sclerotium Poriae Cocoris, Radix Glycyrrhizae, Radix Angelicae Sinensis, Radix Ligustici Wallichii, Radix Conquita Rhemanniae, Radix Astragali Seu Hedysari, Fructus Lycii Chinensis, Cortex Eucommiae, Radix Achyranthis Bidentatae, Radix Dipsaci, Herba Cistanchis, Herba Cynomorii Songarici, Radix Morindae, Tuber Asparagi Cochinensis, Tuber Ophiopogonis Japonicae, Fructus Schizandrae Chinensis, Lignum Aquilariae Agallochae, Pericarpium Citri Reticulatae.

Indications: Tinnitus, weakness of the low back and knees, insomnia, forgetfulness, premature ejaculation, and night sweats. According to Naeser, *Quan Lu Wan* nourishes kidney yin and yang, supplements the *yuan qi*, and nourishes the blood. It is used to treat both yin and yang empty conditions. It treats spermatorrhea and impotence due to either emptiness of kidney yang or yin and also treats various menopathies, such as irregular periods, scanty periods, menorrhagia, and leukorrhea.

Hai Long Bu Wan ★♦
Hai Long Ge Jie Jing ★♦

Ingredients: *Hai Long Bu Wan* are pills composed of Syngnathus, Hippocampus, Testis Capri Hirci, Radix Panacis Ginseng, Radix Angelicae Sinensis, Cortex Cinnamomi, Semen Cuscutae, Radix Alba Paeoniae Lactiflorae, Cortex Radicis Moutan, Herba Dendrobii, Rhizoma Alismatis, Radix Conquita Rehmanniae, Rhizoma Dessicata Zingiberis, and Herba Cum Radice Asari. *Hai Long Ge Jie Jing* is a liquid extract composed of Syngnathus, Gecko, Radix Astragali Seu Hedysari, Radix Panacis Ginseng, Radix Polygoni Multiflori, Radix Angelicae Sinensis, Fructus Lycii Chinensis, and Lignum Aquilariae Agallochae.

Indications: *Hai Long Bu Wan* are indicated for the treatment of emptiness of both qi and blood, premature aging, low back and knee pain, neurasthenia, dizziness due to anemia, weariness and taxation beyond measure, insomnia, and other similar conditions. Fratkin says this medication, because it supplements kidney yang, is also good for impotence and reduced sexual drive in men. He also adds polyuria to its list of indications. *Hai Long Ge Jie Jing* has similar indications to *Hai Long Bu Wan*, such as neurasthenia, weariness and taxation beyond measure, qi and blood dual emptiness, low back and knee pain, loss of strength of the four extremities, dizziness, blurred vision, etc.

Comparison of the Above Formulas

Du Shen Tang is composed of ginseng. Ginseng has the ability to supplement the *yuan qi*, boosting the blood and body fluids, and calm the spirit. It is therefore good for the *xu sun* condition caused by both qi and blood emptiness. However, because ginseng is dry in nature, it can easily enhance the rising of fire. It is therefore not suitable for patients who suffer from fire due to empty yin and is also not suitable for full or *shi* patients. *Du Shen Tang* can be used for rescuing collapsed yang.

Shen Qi Jing is a combination of ginseng and astragalus. Astragalus enhances ginseng's functions of boosting the qi and supplementing the blood. Thus its actions are balanced and therefore its use is safe.

Shen Qi Da Bu Wan is made from both codonopsis and astragalus. Codonopsis' ability to supplement emptiness is not as strong as ginseng's. However, it is also not as dry as ginseng and is, therefore, more balanced. It is more suitable for persons suffering from emptiness of both qi and blood and is also cheaper.

Bei Qi Jing is composed of astragalus and honey. Astragalus boosts the qi, raises yang, and consolidates the *wei qi*. Honey supplements and benefits the body while it also moisturizes. It supplements without being too strong and supplements equally qi and blood in persons with insufficiency of qi and blood.

Zheng Bei Qi Pian and *Bei Qi Jing* are suitable for patients with excessive perspiration due, to emptiness, emptiness edema, nephritis, prolapse of central qi, and other similar conditions. They boost the qi, raise yang, and consolidate the surface.

Shuang Bao Su Kou Fu Ye, *Bei Jing Feng Wang Jing*, *Bei Jing Ling Zhi Feng Wang Jing*, and *Bei Jing Feng Ru Jing Pian* all use ginseng and royal jelly as their ruling ingredients. Royal jelly is an efficacious supplementing medicinal which prevents premature aging. Its moistening ability counteracts ginseng's drying effects. Thus it is suitable for supplementing the elderly.

Honey is a first class herbal medicinal for supplementing and boosting. It can be used for constitutional weakness of the elderly and emptiness weakness of the body. It can be used for a long period of time as a longevity food and is especially good for empty constipation. It is not, however, suitable for patients with diabetes.

Ji Wu Jia Yang Shen Su, Wu Jia Shen Chong Ji, Wu Jia Shen Jing, and *Ji Wu Jia Pian* have similar supplementing and strengthening abilities as does ginseng but at a moderate, lower cost.

He Che Fen is made of human placenta. It contains various human hormones and thus it boosts the body. It is most suitable for the aged, patients suffering from liver diseases, and pulmonary tuberculosis with physical weakness. Because placenta does not possess ginseng's fiery strength, it may be used with persons suffering from empty yin fire. However, because it can injure the stomach/spleen, it should be used only with caution in patients with stomach/spleen emptiness and weakness.

Ling Zhi Qiang Ti Pian is composed of ginseng, ganoderma, and other herbs. It supplements and boosts weakness and debility. It also helps to adjust the nerves.

Yan Nian Yi Suo Jing is for those with constitutional weakness and debility. It helps stop premature aging.

Shi Quan Da Bu Wan (which also can be had as a *gao* or syrup and as a medicated wine) and *Ren Shen Yang Rong Wan* both contain herbal medicinals which supplement the qi and blood. They are suitable for patients with insufficiency of both qi and blood. These medications both supplement the stomach/spleen. Therefore they are very helpful for patients who suffer from

37

emptiness of qi and blood accompanied by poor appetite and poor digestion.

Dang Gui Bu Xue Gao supplements both the qi and blood. It boosts the qi in order to generate the blood. It primarily treats problems associated with emptiness of the blood.

Quan Lu Wan, Hai Long Bu Wan, and *Hai Long Ge Jie Jing* all supplement both the qi and blood. They also assist yang and supplement fire. They are for those with insufficiency of qi and blood and decline of yang who suffer from weak and sore low back and knees, blurred vision, tinnitus, cold extremities, impotence, premature ejaculation, and other similar conditions. These medications are not suitable for those suffering from empty yin fire.

II. Supplementation & Boosting of the Stomach/Spleen

Traditional Chinese Medicine refers to the food one eats as *shui gu* or water and grains. The essence of this *shui gu* is what nourishes the body. The absorption and digestion of water and grains and the transportation and transformation of the essence of *shui gu* to and for the entire body all depend upon the function of the stomach/spleen. Therefore, the health of the human body is strongly related to the quality of stomach/spleen function.

Strong or weak spleen qi refers to strong or weak function of the stomach/spleen. If spleen qi is strong, the appetite is good and one can eat plenty of food with good absorption. The body thence receives good nutrition through the transportation and transformation function of the spleen which thus creates a healthy body with the five *zang* strong and fulfilled. If, on the other hand, spleen qi is weak, one cannot eat or absorb their food well. The whole body, therefore, does not get the nutrients it needs and as a result the whole body becomes weak and the five *zang* fail to store *jing* essence.

Because stomach/spleen function is so important, it is called "the postnatal or Latter Heaven root" and "the source of growth and transformation". The ancients, therefore, always paid great attention to protecting the stomach qi in terms of *yang sheng* or promoting longevity. Likewise, in terms of treating patients in clinical practice, Traditional Chinese Medicine also pays great attention to protecting the stomach qi.

Because the functioning of the *zang fu* in the elderly deteriorates day by day, so does the absorption, transportation, and transformation of the stomach/spleen. Therefore, supplementation of stomach/spleen function in the elderly and the protection of their stomach qi is very important. Below are described the patent medicines which can supplement the spleen and boost the stomach and which can increase the appetite, assist digestion, and therefore improve the nutrition of the body thus making the whole body healthier.

1. Supplementation of the Spleen & Opening the Stomach (*Kai Wei* i.e., whetting the appetite)

Patent medicines used for this purpose have the functions of supplementing the spleen and boosting the qi, increasing the appetite, supplementing nutrition, and thus strengthening the body. Loss of appetite, abdominal bloating after meals, fatigue, pallor, dizziness, loose stools, and other such symptoms mainly develop due to emptiness of spleen qi. Emptiness of spleen qi may sometimes combine with prolapse of middle qi which may then manifest as prolapse of the stomach, uterus, rectum, and other organs.

Si Jun Zi Wan ★◆●

Ingredients: Radix Codonopsis Pilosulae, Rhizoma Atractylodis Macrocephalae, Sclerotium Poriae Cocoris, Radix Glycyrrhizae

Indications: Facial pallor resulting from emptiness of stomach/spleen qi, weakness of the four limbs, feeble voice, loss of appetite, diarrhea, vomiting, a pale tongue with a thin, white coating, and an empty, weak pulse.

Xiang Sha Liu Jun Zi Wan ★◆●

Ingredients: Radix Codonopsis Pilosulae, Sclerotium Poriae Cocoris, Rhizoma Praeparata Pinelliae, Rhizoma Atractylodis Macrocephalae, Radix Glycyrrhizae, Pericarpium Citri Reticulatae, Radix Saussureae Seu Vladimiriae, Fructus Seu Semen Amomi, Rhizoma Recens Zingiberis

Indications: The root of this formula is *Si Jun Zi Tang* discussed above. To it are added orange peel, treated pinellia, saussurea, amomum, and fresh ginger in order to regulate middle qi and harmonize the stomach. These pills are indicated for the treatment of stomach/spleen emptiness and weakness, lack of strength due to emptiness of qi, loss of appetite, abdominal fullness and distention, vomiting, and diarrhea. In addition, Zhu states that this formula is effective for treating burping, regurgitation, stomach gurgling and borborygmus, stomach pain, and chronic diarrhea with a pale face, pale tongue, and a weak or slow pulse and retention of phlegm and dampness due to emptiness of spleen qi.

Jian Pi Wan ★
Ren Shen Jian Pi Wan ★

Ingredients: *Jian Pi Wan* are pills composed of Radix Codonopsis Pilosulae, Fructus Geriminatus Hordei, Rhizoma Atractylodis Macrocephalae, Fructus Immaturus Citri Seu Ponciri, Pericarpium Citri Reticulatae, and Fructus Crataegi. *Ren Shen Jian Pi Wan* is basically the same formula with the substitution of Radix Panacis Ginseng for codonopsis.

Indications: Lack of appetite due to emptiness and weakness of the stomach/spleen, abdominal bloating, and diarrhea. To these, Zhu adds frequently occurring accumulation of food stagnation, low energy, pale face, and a weak pulse as well as frequent diarrhea or loose stools due to dampness associated with emptiness of spleen qi.

Zhi Zhu Wan ★

Ingredients: Fructus Immaturus Citri Seu Ponciri and Rhizoma Atractylodis Macrocephalae

Indications: Lack of appetite and abdominal bloating and distention

Bu Zhong Yi Qi Wan ★◆●

Ingredients: Radix Astragali Seu Hedysari, Radix Codonopsis Pilosulae, Radix Glycyrrhizae, Pericarpium Citri Reticulatae, Rhizoma Cimicifugae, Radix Bupleuri, Rhizoma Atractylodis Macrocephalae, Radix Angelicae Sinensis

Indications: Lack of appetite due to emptiness of stomach/spleen qi, empty perspiration and lethargy, headache, aversion to cold, thirst with a preference to hot drinks,

41

weakness of the four limbs, prolapse of the uterus, rectum, or stomach, chronic diarrhea, and a pale tongue with white coating, and empty, soft, forceless pulse. According to Zhu, *Bu Zhong Yi Qi Wan* also treat chronic, low-grade fever due to emptiness of middle qi with flushing of yang upward.

Comparison of the Above Formulas

Si Jun Zi Wan is the basic formula for supplementing the spleen and boosting the qi. All patients with emptiness of qi may use this formula except those who, due to weak stomach/spleen function, are not able to digest these herbs, in which case one may add orange peel and pinellia to the root formula in order to activate the qi, dry dampness, and open and harmonize the stomach. This then results in *Liu Jun Zi Wan* which is more effective for regulating and harmonizing the stomach/spleen and strengthening digestion.

Xiang Sha Liu Jun Zi Wan adds saussurea and amomum to *Liu Jun Zi Wan* in order to further invigorate the spleen, activate the qi, and open the stomach (i.e., improve the appetite). Not only is it good for improving the digestion and increasing appetite, but it is especially effective for treating abdominal bloating due to emptiness complicated by dampness and stagnant qi.

Jian Pi Wan and *Ren Shen Jian Pi Wan* are both used to strengthen and boost the stomach/spleen, improve the appetite, and stop diarrhea due to stagnant food. These two pills are particularly indicated where dampness and stagnant food complicate emptiness of the stomach/spleen.

Zhi Zhu Wan is used to strengthen the stomach/spleen, improve the appetite, activate the qi, and relieve abdominal bloating due to emptiness of stomach/spleen complicated by predominant stagnant qi.

Bu Zhong Yi Qi Wan is used to strengthen the stomach/spleen and boost the qi as well as promote the arisal of Clear yang. It is mainly used to treat patients with emptiness of stomach/spleen with prolapse of middle qi.

III. Supplementation of the Spleen, Warming the Middle, Arresting Diarrhea, & Soothing Pain

The patent medicines in this category supplement the spleen, boost the qi, eliminate dampness, and stop diarrhea. In addition, they warm the yang and relieve cold, stop abdominal bloating and cold pain, and stop empty cold diarrhea. They are mainly used in patients with emptiness of spleen qi with inhibited spleen transportation and transformation function who suffer from loose stools, loss of appetite, abdominal bloating, a cold feeling in the abdomen, weakness of the four limbs, a flabby tongue, and an empty pulse.

Shen Ling Bai Zhu Wan ★♦●

Ingredients: Semen Dolichoris, Radix Panacis Ginseng, Sclerotium Poriae Cocoris, Rhizoma Atractylodis Macrocephalae, Radix Glycyrrhizae, Radix Dioscoreae Oppositae, Semen Nelumbinis Nuciferae, Radix Platycodi Grandiflori, Fructus Seu Semen Amomi, Semen Coicis Lachryma-jobi

Indications: Diarrhea due to emptiness of stomach/spleen qi with accumulation of dampness, weakness of the four limbs, pallor, poor digestion, fullness in the chest and abdomen, a

43

white, sticky tongue coating, and an empty, slow pulse. According to Naeser, the herbs in this formula are warming but not drying which makes this a particularly gentle prescription for treating digestive disorders. Although this formula is meant to treat spleen qi emptiness with dampness, it can be used when complicated by empty yin.

Fu Zi Li Zhong Wan ★◆●

Ingredients: Radix Panacis Ginseng, Rhizoma Dessicata Zingiberis, Rhizoma Atractylodis Macrocephalae, and Radix Praeparatus Aconiti Carmichaeli

Indications: These pills are indicated for the treatment of empty cold of the stomach/spleen as manifest by a minute pulse, chilling of the four extremities, vomiting, diarrhea, and abdominal pain which desires warmth and pressure. Naeser adds that the pulse may be thin and deep and that the tongue is pale and without much coating. She also includes clear urine in her list of signs and symptoms. Zhu indicates this formula for the treatment of *tai yin* disorders with pronounced internal cold. As for Western medical disease categories, he indicates this prescription for acute gastroenteritis, gastric ulcers, duodenal ulcers, colitis, and gastroptosis all due to cold.

Comparison of the Above Formulas

Shen Ling Bai Zhu Wan is composed of ingredients which supplement the spleen, benefit the qi, stop diarrhea, and leech out dampness. This medicine is, therefore, indicated for patients who suffer from spleen emptiness with inhibition in the spleen's functions of transportation and transformation. This manifests as diarrhea, loose stools, lack of appetite, fatigue, shortness of breath, and a weak pulse with a flabby tongue.

44

Fu Zi Li Zhong Wan not only strengthens and boosts the qi but also warms the middle and disperses cold. It is suitable for empty cold of the middle burner with loose stools, abdominal chilling and pain, loss of appetite, a pale face, minute pulse, chilling of the four limbs, etc. *Sheng Ling Bai Zhu Wan* warmly supplements the middle and eliminates dampness. Whereas, *Fu Zi Li Zhong Wan* warms the middle and disperse cold while supplementing stomach/spleen qi.

IV. Supplementation of the Kidneys & Strengthening Yang

Strengthening yang means to supplement and boost kidney yang and also to warm and supplement the *ming men zhi huo* or the fire of the gate of life. But what are kidney yang and life fire? These are the source of warmth and the original spring of strength. Emptiness of kidney yang results in the body suffering from internal cold and yin. Thus kidney yang is considered the source of body warmth. It warms the *zang* and *fu* and increases their activity as well as all the physical functions of the entire body. In terms of yang, fire and qi have the same function which is to increase the body's physical activities. A decrease in the body's fire makes the body vulnerable to attack by external cold. This manifests in such complaints as cold limbs, fatigue, cold and painful low back and knees, frequent urination, and decreased sex drive. If this situation becomes more severe, it will manifest as premature ejaculation or impotence in men and cold uterus and infertility in women.

Kidney yin and kidney yang are both mutually interdependent and intersupporting. As it is said, "Decline of yin reaches yang" and "Decline of yang reaches yin". Typically, kidney yang emptiness results from kidney yin emptiness. However, on occasion, it is also possible that kidney yang emptiness may develop into kidney yin emptiness. It is therefore a rule that when supplementing kidney yang, one also must supplement kidney yin as well.

As people age, their kidney *jing* becomes overtaxed and kidney yang becomes empty. Thus, in strengthening the elderly, we need to supplement the kidneys and strengthen the yang. This is also true in the case of younger people who have prematurely lost their kidney *jing* due to too much sex, and the same methods may be applied to strengthen their bodies as well.

Generally speaking, all kidney yang herbal medicinals are warm or hot and, therefore, strengthen fire. Consequently, caution must be taken when using this class of ingredient in patients with empty yin fire and especially when using ginseng and deer antler.

Jin Gui Shen Qi Wan ★◆●

Ingredients: Radix Conquita Rehmanniae, Radix Dioscoreae Oppositae, Sclerotium Poriae Cocoris, Fructus Corni Officinalis, Cortex Radicis Moutan, Rhizoma Alismatis, Cortex Cinnamomi, and Radix Praeparatus Aconiti Carmichaeli

Indications: Lumbar pain with weak knees due to emptiness of kidney yang, sensations of cold in the lower half of the body, abdominal spasm and pain, insomnia, restlessness, difficulty in and frequency of urination, a flabby, pale tongue, and an empty, weak pulse which is deep and weak in the *chi* or foot position.

You Gui Wan ★

Ingredients: Radix Conquita Rehmanniae, Radix Praeparatus Aconiti Carmichaeli, Cortex Cinnamomi, Fructus Corni Officinalis, Fructus Lycii Chinensis, Radix Dioscoreae Oppositae, Cortex Eucommiae Ulmoidis, Radix Angelicae Sinensis, Semen Cuscutae, and Gelatinum Cornu Cervi

Indications: Fatigue due to insufficiency of kidney yang, loss of appetite, aversion to cold, and incontinence of urine. In addition, these pills treat spontaneous perspiration, premature ejaculation, impotence, low back and knee pain and soreness, dizziness, and spermatorrhea. The tongue is pale and the pulse is deep, slow, and weak.

Gui Lin Ji ★♦

Ingredients: Cornu Cervi Parvum, Fructus Psoraleae Corylifoliae, Semen Impatientis, Herba Cum Radice Asari, Radix Rehmanniae, Cortex Eucommiae Ulmoidis, Halitum, Flos Caryophylli, Periostracum Bombycis, Dragonfly, Radix Conquita Rehmanniae, Herba Cistanchis, Cortex Radicis Lycii, Radix Praeparatus Aconiti Carmichaeli, Tuber Asparagi Cochinensis, Radix Dioscoreae Oppositae, Radix Glycyrrhizae, Squama Manitis, Fructus Lycii Chinensis, Herba Cynomorii, Herba Epimedii, Fructus Seu Semen Amomi, Radix Achyranthis Bidentatae, Semen Cuscutae, Hippocampus, Sulphur, Cinnabaris

Indications: Emptiness of both qi and blood, impotence, premature ejaculation due to emptiness of *ming men* fire, kidney cold/*jing* chilled, yin cold abdominal pain, tinnitus, sweating, insomnia, etc.

47

Shen Rong Pian ★♦

Ingredients: Radix Panacis Ginseng and Cornu Cervi Parvum

Indications: Constitutional emptiness and fear of chill, fatigue, weakness of the low back and knees, impotence, and premature ejaculation

Ren Shen Lu Rong Wan ★♦

Ingredients: Radix Panacis Ginseng, Cornu Cervi Parvum, Herba Cistanchis, Semen Cuscutae, Radix Morindae, Sclerotium Poriae Cocoris, Radix Angelicae Sinensis, Arillus Euphoriae Longanae, Cortex Eucommiae Ulmoidis, Radix Achyranthis Bidentatae, Fructus Psoraleae Corylifoliae, Fructus Schizandrae Chinensis, Fructus Lycii Chinensis, etc.

Indications: Constitutional emptiness after disease, weakness of the low back and knees, insomnia, forgetfulness, dizziness, sweating due to emptiness of yin, lack of appetite, etc.

Shen Rong Wan ★

Ingredients: Radix Panacis Ginseng, Cornu Cervi Parvum, Fructus Lycii Chinensis, Herba Cistanchis, Radix Polygalae Tenuifoliae, Semen Cuscutae, Radix Astragali Seu Hedysari, Tuber Asparagi Cochinensis, Tuber Ophiopogonis Japonicae, Cortex Eucommiae Ulmoidis, Fructus Psoraleae Corylifoliae, Radix Polygoni Multiflori, Fructus Corni Officinalis, Bulbus Fritillariae, Cortex Cinnamomi, Fructus Foeniculi, etc.

Indications: Soreness and pain of the low back and knees, insomnia, forgetfulness, perspiration due to either empty yin or yang, decrease in visual acuity, impotence, premature ejaculation, dizziness, and tinnitus

Ren Shen Wai Sheng Wan ★

Ingredients: Radix Panacis Ginseng, Cornu Cervi Parvum, Herba Cistanchis, Arillus Euphoriae Longanae, Herba Cynomorii, Radix Polygoni Multiflori, Succinum, Fructus Zizyphi Spinosae, Radix Angelicae Sinensis, Cortex Eucommiae Ulmoidis, etc.

Indications: All emptinesses and one hundred weaknesses (i.e., emptiness and debility of all kinds), weakness of the low back and knees, weakness of the four limbs, fatigue, loss of appetite, forgetfulness, insomnia, dizziness, blurring of vision, and night sweats due to empty yin

Dong Bei San Bao Jiu ★

Ingredients: Radix Panacis Ginseng, Cornu Cervi Parvum, Marten's penis

Indications: General kidney yang weakness symptoms, impotence, premature ejaculation, weakness of the low back and knees, cold, damp scrotum, and other such conditions

Shen Rong Bian Wan ★♦

Ingredients: Radix Panacis Ginseng, Cornu Cervi Parvum, Marten's penis, Hippocampus, Cortex Eucommiae Ulmoidis, Fructus Lycii Chinensis, Cortex Cinnamomi, etc.

Indications: Emptiness and decline of kidney qi, weakness and decline of the nerves, impotence, premature ejaculation, and other such symptoms of kidney emptiness in both men and women

49

Zhi Bao San Bian Jing ★♦
Zhi Bao San Bian Wan ★♦

Ingredients: Available as both a liquid extract and as pills, these patent medicines contain Radix Panacis Ginseng, Radix Astragali Seu Hedysari, Cornu Cervi Parvum, Hippocampus, Cortex Cinnamomi, Lignum Aquilariae Agallochae, Radix Morindae, Herba Epimedii, Testis Et Penis Otoriae, deer testicles and penis, dog testicles and penis, Fructus Corni Officinalis, Radix Polygoni Multiflori, Radix Dioscoreae Oppositae, Cortex Eucommiae Ulmoidis, Radix Polygalae Tenuifoliae, Semen Plantaginis, Cortex Phellodendri, Fructus Psoraleae Corylifoliae, Os Draconis, Fructus Foeniculi, Cortex Radicis Moutan, Radix Angelicae Sinensis, Radix Alba Paeoniae Lactiflorae, etc.

Indications: Constitutional weakness, emptiness, and decline, premature aging and debility, decline and weakness of the nerves, weakness of the low back and knees, anemia, dizziness, heart palpitations due to weakness and decline, forgetfulness, spontaneous and empty sweating, cold stomach, facial pallor, lack of appetite due to emptiness of qi, no strength in the four extremities, blood emptiness in women, senile asthma, etc. Naeser says this formula nourishes both *jing* and blood, strengthens the qi, and increases the function of the brain. Zhu says that it is effective in treating impotence and spermatorrhea.

San Bian Jiu ★

Ingredients: This medicinal wine or tincture is composed of essentially the same ingredients as the above extract and pills.

Indications: Same as above

Bu Sheng Jiao Nan aka *Nan Bao* ★

Ingredients: Donkey kidneys, pig kidneys, Hippocampus, Gelatinum Asini, Radix Astragali Seu Hedysari, Fructus Corni Officinalis, etc.

Indications: Kidney yang emptiness and weakness, impotence, premature ejaculation, weakness of the low back and knees, scrotum damp and chilly, essence spirit taxation, loss of appetite, and other such conditions

Jin Suo Gu Jing Wan ★◆●

Ingredients: Semen Euryalis, Stamen Nelumbinis Nuciferae, calcined Os Draconis, calcined Concha Ostreae, Semen Nelumbinis Nuciferae, Semen Astragali Complanati

Indications: Premature ejaculation due to emptiness of the kidneys not consolidating or holding *jing* essence, fatigue, weakness of the four limbs, low back pain, tinnitus, pale tongue with white coating, and a fine, weak pulse

Comparison of the Above Formulas

Jin Gui Shen Qi Wan and *You Gui Wan* are typical patent medicines for warming the *ming men* fire. These medicines can be used for decline of *ming men* fire with such symptoms as coldness of the lower half of the body and low energy as well as long, clear polyuria. They are suitable for treating diabetes, general kidney diseases, and enlarged prostate glands in the elderly.

Gui Lin Ji is known for its function of boosting *ming men* fire and nourishing the qi and blood. It is used for patients

51

suffering from constitutional emptiness and weakness, impotence and premature ejaculation due to decline of *ming men* fire, cold kidneys/chilly *jing*, chilly pain of the low back, blurred vision, tinnitus, etc.

Shen Rong Pian, Ren Shen Lu Rong Wan, Shen Rong Wan, Shen Rong Wai Sheng Wan, Zhi Bei San Bao Jiu, Shen Rong Bian Wan, etc. all contain ginseng which greatly supplements *yuan qi* and Cornu Cervi Parvum which supplements kidney yang, fills the *jing*, and nourishes the blood. All of these medicines can be used for kidney emptiness and yang weakness with impotence, premature ejaculation, low back soreness and pain, fatigue, lack of strength, fear of cold, chilled limbs, dizziness, blurred vision, and other such symptoms of bodily emptiness and decline.

Jin Suo Gu Jing Wan supplements the kidneys and astringes the essence. It is for the treatment of spermatorrhea and premature ejaculation due to decline and weakness of the kidneys' ability to hold and consolidate.

V. Moistening Yin & Supplementation of the Kidneys, Subduing Fire & Decreasing Heat

The kidneys are the *zang* organ which store the *jing* essence. Moistening yin means moistening and supplementing kidney *jing*. Kidney *jing* rules the growth of the human body during youth. Sufficiency of kidney *jing qi* makes for strong reproductive function. However, during the aging process, the body's kidney *jing* is weakened thus diminishing one's sexual ability and reproductive capacity.

Likewise, our bones, bone marrow, teeth, and hair all have a close relationship with kidney *jing*. Sufficient kidney *jing* results in strong bones, healthy teeth, healthy bone marrow for good memory, and a full head of healthy hair. Again, because kidney *jing* is inevitably consumed and becomes deficient during aging, one's low back and knees become weak, one's teeth become loose, and one may experience vertigo, tinnitus and deafness, slowed responses, poor memory, forgetfulness, and loss of hair.

Additionally, emptiness of kidney yin may give rise to internal heat and fire. This, in turn, may cause night sweats, bone steaming heat, heat in the center of the hands and feet, thirst with desire to drink, a dry, sore throat, restlessness, irritability, a red tongue, and rapid pulse.

The various patent medicines described below all moisten and supplement kidney yin, subdue fire, and decrease heat. Some of them are also good for supplementing emptiness of *jing* essence. These medications are suitable for patients with stirring of empty yin fire causing liver disease, hypertension, diabetes, hyperthyroidism, kidney disease, and tuberculosis.

Liu Wei Di Huang Wan ★◆●
Zhi Bai Di Huang Wan ★◆●

Ingredients: Radix Conquita Rehmanniae, Fructus Corni Officinalis, Radix Dioscoreae Oppositae, Sclerotium Poriae Cocoris, Rhizoma Alismatis, Cortex Radicis Moutan. The ingredients in *Zhi Bai Di Huang Wan* are the same as those above plus the addition of Rhizoma Anemarrhenae and Cortex Phellodendri.

Indications: Kidney yin emptinessess, flaring upward of empty fire, soreness and weakness of the low back and knees, dizziness, vertigo, tinnitus and deafness, premature ejaculation, diabetes, bone steaming heat, heat in the center of the hands and feet, loss of teeth, dribbling urination, a red tongue with scant coating, and a thready, rapid pulse. *Zhi Bai Di Huang Wan* are indicated when empty fire is more pronounced.

Da Bu Yin Wan ★♦

Ingredients: Rhizoma Anemarrhenae, Cortex Phellodendri, Radix Conquita Rehmanniae, Plastrum Testudinis, pig's spinal marrow

Indications: Bone steaming heat, night sweats, cough with hemoptysis, epistaxis, restlessness, a red tongue with scant coating, and a *chi* or foot position pulse which is fast and forceful

He Che Da Zao Wan ★♦

Ingredients: Plastrum Testudinis, Radix Conquita Rehmanniae, Radix Codonopsis Pilosulae, Cortex Phellodendri, Cortex Eucommiae Ulmoidis, Placenta Hominis, Radix Achyranthis Bidentatae, Tuber Asparagi Cochinensis, Tuber Ophiopogonis Japonicae, Sclerotium Poriae Cocoris, Fructus Seu Semen Amomi

Indications: Liver/kidney emptiness and weakness resulting in emptiness injury manifesting as weakness of the low back and knees, bone-steaming heat, nocturnal emissions, and similar such conditions

Qi Bao Mei Xu Dan ★

Ingredients: Radix Polygoni Multiflori, Radix Achyranthis Bidentatae, Semen Cuscutae, Radix Angelicae Sinensis, Fructus Psoraleae Corylifoliae, Fructus Lycii Chinensis, Sclerotium Poriae Cocoris

Indications: Decline and weakness of kidney water and qi and blood insufficiency resulting in premature graying of the hair, loosened teeth, spermatorrhea, and bones and sinews without strength

Shou Wu Pian ★◆

Ingredients: Radix Polygoni Multiflori

Indications: Emptiness of blood and bodily debility, dizziness, tinnitus, and weakness of the low back and knees

Yu Quan Wan ★◆

Ingredients: Radix Trichosanthis Kirlowii, Radix Rehmanniae, Fructus Schizandrae Chinensis, Radix Puerariae Lobatae, Radix Glycyrrhizae

Indications: Nourishes kidney yin, clears empty heat, relieves thirst due to depleted kidney yin, and promotes salivation. These pills are used to treat yin depletion and damaged body fluids and mild to moderate diabetes.

Comparison of the Above Formulas

Liu Wei Di Huang Wan and *Zhi Bai Di Huang Wan* both moisten yin and supplement the kidneys as well as subdue empty fire. For the latter purpose, *Zhi Bai Di Huang Wan* is more effective. Both treat dizziness, tinnitus, dry mouth, steaming-bone heat, night sweats and other such conditions due to emptiness and weakness of kidney yin.

Da Bu Yin Wan moistens yin and clears internal heat. It is indicated for the treatment of perspiration and bleeding due to

55

internal heat in turn due to emptiness of yin, steaming-bone heat, palpitations, and a red tongue with scant coating.

He Che Da Zao Wan moistens and supplements kidney yin, subdues heat, and consolidates the essence. It is indicated for the treatment of kidney essence decline and weakness causing weakness of the low back and knees, steaming-bone heat, and spermatorrhea.

Qi Bao Mei Xu Dan and *Shou Wu Pian* both supplement *jing* essence and blood. Their power of subduing fire is not very strong. Rather they primarily treat conditions due to decline and weakness of *jing* and blood, such as premature greying of the hair, loosened teeth, and lack of strength of the sinews and bones.

Yu Quan Wan is indicated for the treatment of diabetes.

VI. Supplementation of the Kidneys, Supplementation of the Heart, Strengthening the Brain, & Calming the Spirit

In Traditional Chinese Medicine, the brain is closely related to three *zang:* the kidneys, the heart, and the liver. The kidneys store the *jing* essence and it is the *jing* which produces the bone marrow which in turn is stored in the brain. Thus it can be said that the transformation and generation of the brain is dependent upon the bone marrow which is dependent upon kidney *jing*. When kidney *jing* is sufficient, brain function is increased and consciousness is clear, response to stimuli is quick, and the memory is good. As one ages, *yuan qi* becomes insufficient and thus kidney *jing* becomes deficient as well. This manifests as retardation of brain function and leads to such symptoms as forgetfulness and slow response. To rectify this situation, it is necessary to administer medicines which supplement the kidneys, boost the *jing*, and strengthen the brain.

The heart controls the spirit and the will. It also controls consciousness and mental function. If the heart maintains its healthy function, qi and blood are then sufficient and one will have a clear mind, abundant energy, and healthy sleeping habits. If healthy heart function declines due to a decrease in heart qi and blood, evil heat will accumulate in the heart and phlegm fluids will disturb the heart spirit. This may give rise to palpitations, sleeplessness, irregular heart beat, and other such conditions. Because qi becomes empty and blood becomes scant in the elderly, the heart spirit is not nourished and phlegm heat tends to accumulate. For these problems it is necessary to administer medicinals which nourish the heart and calm the spirit.

The liver stores the blood and is related to the emotional aspect of the individual. If the liver fails to store sufficient blood or if one is overtaxed by emotions such as depression or anger, then symptoms such as irritability, palpitations, and insomnia will occur. Because in Chinese medicine *jing* essence and blood can mutually transform into one another, supplementation of the kidneys also supplements the liver. Similarly, when nourishing heart blood, liver blood is also nourished. Thus the same method of supplementation accomplishes both ends. In addition, liver depression and qi stagnation can also disturb the heart spirit and for this medicinals which smoothe the liver and relieve depression should be used.

1. Nourishing the Heart, Calming the Spirit

The patent medicines described below boost heart qi and nourish heart blood. In addition, they nourish and supplement heart yin and subdue heart fire. Some of them are also indicated for the treatment of weakness and emptiness of both qi and blood not nourishing heart spirit, heart yin insufficiency, and empty fire disturbing heart spirit.

Bu Xin Dan aka *Tian Wang Bu Xin Dan* ★◆●

Ingredients: Radix Panacis Ginseng, Sclerotium Poriae Cocoris, Radix Scrophulariae Ningpoensis, Tuber Ophiopogonis Japonicae, Tuber Asparagi Cochinensis, Radix Salviae Miltorrhizae, Radix Angelicae Sinensis, Semen Biotae Orientalis, Radix Polygalae Tenuifoliae, Fructus Schizandrae Chinensis, Semen Zizyphi Spinosae, Radix Platycodi Grandiflori, Radix Rehmanniae

Indications: Heart organ diseases, neurasthenia, hyperthyroid symptoms with irritable palpitations, insomnia, fatigue, forgetfulness, dry stools, sores in the mouth and on the tongue, a red tongue with scant coating, and a fine, rapid pulse

Gui Pi Wan ★◆●

Ingredients: Radix Panacis Ginseng, Semen Zizyphi Spinosae, Radix Astragali Seu Hedysari, Radix Saussureae Seu Vladimiriae, Rhizoma Atractylodis Macrocephalae, Rhizoma Cyperi Rotundi, Sclerotium Poriae Cocoris, Pericarpium Citri Reticulatae, Radix Angelicae Sinensis, Radix Polygalae Tenuifoliae, Radix Glycyrrhizae. It should be noted that this version of *Gui Pi Wan* is somewhat different from that given in other texts. It does not contain longans and does contain both citrus and cyperus which are not in the pill versions of this famous formula as described by Zhu or Naeser.

Indications: Neurasthenia accompanied by palpitations, insomnia, forgetfulness, dream-disturbed sleep, loss of appetite, facial pallor and sallowness, a pale tongue with a thin, white coating, and a thready, weak pulse.

Bai Zi Yang Xin Wan ★♦

Ingredients: Semen Biotae Orientalis, Radix Astragali Seu Hedysari, Sclerotium Poriae Cocoris, Radix Ligustici Wallichii, Semen Zizyphi Spinosae, Radix Angelicae Sinensis, Fructus Schizandrae Chinensis, Rhizoma Pinelliae Ternatae, Radix Polygalae Tenuifoliae, Radix Glycyrrhizae, Radix Codonopsis Pilosulae, Cortex Cinnamomi

Indications: Difficulty concentrating due to insufficiency of heart qi, restlessness, insomnia, and forgetfulness

Shen Jing Shuai Rou Wan ★♦

Ingredients: Raw Magnetitum, Caulis Polygoni Multiflori, Flos Albizziae Julibrissinis, Radix Salviae Miltorrhizae, Rhizoma Polygonati, Semen Zizyphi Spinosae, Bulbus Fritillariae, Radix Angelicae Sinensis, Radix Polygalae Tenuifoliae, Fructus Schizandrae Chinensis

Indications: Insomnia, dizziness, heart palpitations, bodily weariness, and tinnitus

An Shen Bu Xin Pian ★♦

Ingredients: Radix Salviae Miltorrhizae, Herba Ecliptae, Radix Rehmanniae, Caulis Polygoni Multiflori, Fructus Ligustri Lucidi, Fructus Schizandrae Chinensis, Semen Cuscutae, etc.

Indications: Dizziness, insomnia, palpitations, restlessness, tinnitus, and forgetfulness due to insufficiency of yin and blood

Yang Xue An Shen Pian ★

Ingredients: Herba Agrimoniae, Herba Ecliptae, Caulis Polygoni Multiflori, Cortex Albizziae Julibrissinis, Caulis Milletiae Jixueteng, Radix Conquita Rehmanniae, Radix Rehmanniae

Indications: Insomnia, forgetfulness, dream-disturbed sleep, empty kidney soreness of the low back, dizziness, and fatigue

Ling Zhi Pian ★♦

Ingredients: Fructificatio Ganodermae Lucidae

Indications: Neurasthenia, coronary heart disease, chronic bronchitis, etc.

Zhu Sha An Shen Wan ★●

Ingredients: Cinnabaris, Rhizoma Coptidis, Radix Angelicae Sinensis, Radix Rehmanniae, Radix Glycyrrhizae

Indications: Insomnia, heart fire flaring upward, injury of yin and blood causing restlessness of heart spirit, palpitation, heartburn, insomnia or dream-disturbed sleep, a red tongue, and a fine, rapid pulse

Zheng Jing An Mian Wan ★

Ingredients: Semen Zizyphi Spinosae, Radix Polygalae Tenuifoliae, Sclerotium Poriae Cocoris, Fructus Gardeniae Jasminoidis, Radix Glycyrrhizae, Massa Medica Fermentata

Indications: Heart emptiness with heat, restlessness and insomnia, dream-disturbed sleep, fatigue, and neurasthenia

Sheng Mai Yin ★

Ingredients: This liquid extract is composed of Radix Panacis Ginseng, Tuber Ophiopogonis Japonicae, Fructus Schizandrae Chinensis.

Indications: Palpitations and shortness of breath caused by injury to both the qi and yin, a minute, empty pulse, dry mouth and throat, a chronic cough which has injured the lungs, injury to both the qi and yin, a dry cough and shortness of breath, spontaneous perspiration, and shock

Long Yan Rou ★♦

Arillus Euphoriae Longanae or longans are a very healthy food which are nourishing and supplementing. Traditional Chinese Medicine believes that longans boost the spleen and increase (literally lengthen) one's wisdom. It is said of them that they "open the stomach (i.e., improve the appetite) and boost the spleen, supplement one's spirit and increase one's wisdom". Longans are suitable for the treatment of insomnia due to emptiness and weakness of the body, overthinking, lack of appetite, etc. For this purpose, 10 grams each of longans and Semen Zizyphi Spinosae can be decocted in water and drunk. For emptiness and weakness of the stomach/spleen, loss of appetite, and diarrhea, decoct 10 grams of longans with 3 slices of fresh ginger in water and take once per day. For anemia, take 5 grams of longans, 15 grams of Semen Nelumbinis Nuciferae, and 30 grams of polished glutinous rice, decoct into a gruel and take once per day. Because this food is warm, hot, and dry, it should not be used by persons who have empty yin with heat, epistaxis, etc. It should also not be used in patients with cough and excessive phlegm.

Comparison of the Above Formulas

Bu Xin Dan is a supplementing medicinal for the qi, blood, and yin which is used to treat heart emptiness and insufficiency which in turn cause heart spirit not being calm. In addition, it also treats emptiness of yin with flaring fire accompanied by dry stools, a red tongue with scant coating, etc.

Gui Pi Wan and *Bai Zi Yang Xin Wan* are good for boosting heart qi and nourishing heart blood. They are appropriate for empty qi/scant blood conditions causing the heart spirit not to be calm and, therefore, restlessness, palpitations, and insomnia. In particular, *Gui Pi Wan* supplements both the heart and spleen in cases where the heart spirit is not calm and there is emptiness of the spleen with decreased appetite, etc.

Shen Jing Shuai Rou Wan, An Shen Bu Xin Pian, and *Yang Xue An Shen Pian* are all used to moisten yin, nourish the blood, and calm the *shen*. They are all indicated for insufficiency of yin and blood with empty fire manifesting as heart palpitations, less sleep and more dreams, restlessness, dizziness, tinnitus, and other such conditions.

Ling Zhi Pian is a general tonic which calms the *shen* and also can be used in the treatment of chronic bronchitis.

Zhu Sha An Shen Wan and *Zheng Jing An Mian Wan* are both medications for nourishing heart blood and clearing heart fire. They are used to treat heart emptiness with heat and to calm the heart spirit in cases of insomnia and dream-disturbed sleep, and palpitations in the center of the chest with a red tongue and a fine, rapid pulse.

Sheng Mai Yin supplements both the qi and yin in cases where qi and yin have been injured and there are heart palpitations and shortness of breath with a minute pulse and excessive perspiration and similar conditions due to constitutional emptiness and weakness of the body.

2. Supplementation of the Kidneys & Strengthening the Brain

The patent medicines described below all supplement the kidneys and boost the *jing*, strengthen the brain and the wisdom, intelligence, or memory. They are used for patients who suffer from emptiness of *yuan qi* causing kidney *jing* taxation and deficiency with such symptoms as decreased memory, slow response, dizziness, tinnitus, palpitations, and insomnia.

Nao Ling Shu ★

Ingredients: Radix Panacis Ginseng, Cornu Cervi Parvum, Plastrum Testudinis, Gelatinum Plastri Testudinis, Gelatinum Cornu Cervi, Sclerotium Pararadicis Poriae Cocoris, Fructus Schizandrae Chinensis, Fructus Lycii Chinensis, Fructus Xanthii, Herba Epimedii, Radix Conquita Rehmanniae, Tuber Ophiopogonis Japonicae, Rhizoma Polygonati, Radix Polygalae Tenuifoliae, fried Semen Zizyphi Spinosae, Fructus Zizyphi Jujubae, white sugar

63

Indications: Neurasthenia, headache and dizziness, forgetfulness and insomnia, and tinnitus

Bu Nao Wan ★♦

Ingredients: Radix Angelicae Sinensis, Semen Zizyphi Spinosae, Fructus Schizandrae Chinensis, Fructus Lycii Chinensis, Succinum, Tuber Gastrodiae Elatae, Dens Draconis, Radix Polygalae Tenuifoliae, Semen Biotae Orientalis, Rhizoma Praeparata Cum Fellem Bovis Arisaematis, Rhizoma Acori Graminei, Semen Juglandis, Herba Cistanchis

Indications: Neurasthenia, decreased memory, restlessness, and physical fatigue

Jian Nao Bu Shen Wan ★♦

Ingredients: Radix Panacis Ginseng, Sclerotium Poriae Cocoris, Fructus Seu Semen Amomi, Cornu Cervi Parvum, Semen Zizyphi Spinosae, Cinnabaris, Cortex Cinnamomi, Cortex Eucommiae Ulmoidis, Radix Polygalae Tenuifoliae, and an additional unspecified twelve ingredients

Indications: Kidneys empty, body weak, neurasthenia, insomnia, dizziness, tinnitus, and other such similar conditions

VII. Supplementation & Boosting of the Liver & Kidneys, Strengthening the Low Back & Knees

The liver governs the sinews and the kidneys rule the bones. The low back or lumbus is the mansion of the kidneys. Therefore, low back pain and lack of strength in the legs and knees are often related to the two organs, the liver and kidneys. During the aging process, kidney *jing* becomes empty and liver blood becomes insufficient to nourish the sinews. This then results in low back pain.

Low back and knee pain due to emptiness is divided into two types: empty yin and empty yang. Lumbar and knee pain due to emptiness of yang is accompanied by symptoms such as shortness of breath, fatigue, cold limbs, facial pallor, frequent urination, a pale tongue, and deep pulse. Lumbar pain due to emptiness of yin, on the other hand, is accompanied by such symptoms as dry mouth, dry throat, restlessness, insomnia, dizziness, tinnitus, heat in the centers of the hands and feet, a red tongue, and a fast pulse. The elderly typically suffer from emptiness of both yin and yang.

Jian Bu Hu Qian Wan ★

Ingredients: Cortex Phellodendri, Pericarpium Citri Reticulatae, Plastrum Testudinis, Rhizoma Dessicata Zingiberis, Bulbus Fritillariae, Radix Conquita Rehmanniae, Radix Alba Paeoniae Lactiflorae, Herba Cynomorii, Os Tigridis

Indications: Soreness and pain in the knees and low back due to emptiness of liver/kidney yin, sinews and bones withered and wobbly, knees and legs flaccid and weak, difficulty walking, a red tongue with scant coating, and a fine, weak pulse

Jian Yao Wan ★

Ingredients: Cortex Eucommiae Ulmoidis, Fructus Psoraleae Corylifoliae, Bulbus Allii, Semen Juglandis

Indications: Sore low back due to kidney deficiency, dizziness, tinnitus, dribbling urination, etc.

Yao Tong Pian ★◆

Ingredients: Cortex Eucommiae Ulmoidis, Olibanum, Radix Achyranthis Bidentatae, Eupolyphagae Seu Opisthoplatiae, Radix Angelicae Sinensis, Radix Dipsaci, etc. Naeser lists the additional ingredients as Rhizoma Cibotti Barometz, Rhizoma Atractylodis Macrocephalae, and Fructus Psoraleae Corylifoliae. According to Zhu, there are at least two different versions of this formula.

Indications: Kidney emptiness low back pain, low back and muscular strain and weakness and other such conditions

Hu Gu Shen Rong Jiu ★

Ingredients: Radix Panacis Ginseng, Cornu Cervi Parvum, Os tigridis, Os Leopardis, Rhizoma Dioscoreae Nipponicae, Flos Carthami, Radix Astragali Seu Hedysari, Radix Angelicae Sinensis, Radix Ligustici Wallichii, Radix Aconiti Caowu, Rhizoma Polygonati Odorati, Radix Achyranthis Bidentatae, Radix Conquita Rehmanniae, Olibanum, Myrrha

Indications: Lack of strength in the low back and knees due to deficiency of both qi and blood, wind cold damp *bi* of the upper and lower extremities, sinew and bone soreness and pain

Du Zhong Hu Gu Jiu ★

Ingredients: The ingredients in this medicinal wine are Cortex Eucommiae Ulmoidis, Os tigridis, Zaocys Dhumnades, Radix Panacis Ginseng, Radix Pseudoginseng, Radix Angelicae Sinensis, Radix Ligustici Wallichii, Fructus Chaenomelis Lagenariae, Herba Aristolochiae, Radix Clematidis Chinensis, Ramus Photiniae, Caulis Milletiae Jixueteng, etc.

Indications: Lack of strength of the sinews and bones, difficulty walking, soreness and pain of the low back and knees, wind damp pain of the low back and legs

Gu Zhe Zeng Sheng Pian ★♦

Ingredients: Radix Conquita Rehmanniae, Rhizoma Recens Zingiberis, Herba Cistanchis, Herba Epimedii, Herba Pyrolae. Ginger seems to be a typographical error in the main text. Zhu discusses a similar formula, *Kang Gu Zeng Sheng Pian*, the ingredients of which include in addition to the above: Radix Dioscoreae, Herba Geranii, Caulis Et Folium Hederae, Fructus Liquidambaris Taiwanianae, and Os Tigridis.

Indications: Hyperplasia of the bone, i.e., bone spurs and osteophytes. Zhu states that *Kang Gu Zeng Sheng Pian* is especially good for strengthening the sinews and bones and relieving pain in the elderly.

Comparison of the Above Formulas

Jian Bu Hu Qian Wan is used to supplement the kidneys and liver and to strengthen the sinews and bone in cases of liver/kidney deficiency and weakness causing difficulty in walking.

Jian Yao Wan is used to supplement the kidneys and strengthen the low back. It is indicated for low back soreness and pain due to kidney emptiness. It also treats lack of strength in the low back and legs.

Yao Tong Pian is used to supplement the kidneys and strengthen the low back and also to activate the blood and stop pain. It treats low back pain due to emptiness of the kidneys and low back muscular soreness and weakness, injury due to

67

twisting, and other similar conditions.

Hu Gu Shen Rong Jiu and *Du Zhong Hu Gu Jiu* both supplement the kidneys and boost the qi. They treat wind dampness and stop soreness and pain. In addition, they treat soreness and pain of the low back and legs due to constitutional emptiness, lack of strength of the sinews and bones, and flaccidity conditions. They are also appropriate for the treatment of wind damp pain of the low back and legs.

Gu Zhe Zeng Sheng Pian supplements and boosts the liver and kidneys. It nourishes the blood and supplements the *jing*. Therefore, it treats osteophytes and articular hyperplasia in the elderly.

VIII. Supplementation of the Kidneys, Suppressing Yang, & Improving Hearing

The elderly typically suffer from decrease in auditory acuity, hardness of hearing, and deafness. Traditional Chinese Medicine says that the ears are the orifice of the kidneys and, therefore, many conditions of the ears and hearing are related to the kidneys. However, since the liver and kidneys are so closely related, a good doctor needs to spend some time to find the root problem causing disturbance of the hearing. Even the spleen can be related to hearing problems, and it is necessary to divide hearing problems into emptiness and fullness as well.

Emptiness patterns are mainly associated with kidney *jing* deficiency and weakness, yin emptiness, and yang floating upward. On occasion, this condition may also occur due to emptiness and decline of the stomach/spleen. Patients with this type of hearing impairment will have tinnitus, dizziness, vertigo, soreness of the low back and legs, palpitations, and weak, forceless pulse. In such cases, it is necessary to treat by nourishing and moistening kidney yin and levelling and suppressing floating yang.

Fullness patterns result from fullness of liver/gallbladder fire rising up. This causes distention in the head and headache, vexation, dry stools, yellow urine, and slippery, wiry, forceful pulse. In this case, it is necessary to clear and subdue liver fire and level and envelope liver yang.

Tinnitus usually precedes the development of deafness. Therefore this symptom should not be left untreated. In the elderly it is usually due to the decline of the kidneys and *jing qi* insufficiency. It should be treated primarily by supplementing the kidneys and boosting the *jing*. In the elderly, kidney *jing* deficiency is the leading cause of tinnitus and deafness.

Ci Zhu Wan ★◆

Ingredients: Magnetitum, Cinnabaris, Massa Medica Fermentata

Indications: Palpitations, insomnia, tinnitus, deafness, and blurred vision

Er Long Zuo Ci Wan ★◆

Ingredients: Radix Conquita Rehmanniae, Radix Dioscoreae Oppositae, Fructus Corni Officinalis, Sclerotium Poriae Cocoris, Rhizoma Alismatis, Cortex Radicis Moutan, Fructus Schizandrae Chinensis, Magnetitum

Indications: Tinnitus, deafness, insomnia, and other similar conditions due to liver/kidney insufficiency.

69

Comparison of the Above Formulas

Ci Zhu Wan is indicated for both supplementing kidney *jing* and suppressing and enveloping yang. It treats liver/kidney deficiency and weakness, *jing* and blood insufficiency, and empty yang floating upward causing tinnitus and deafness as well as empty vexation insomnia. In addition, it also treats blurred vision.

Er Long Zuo Ci Wan supplements liver/kidney essence and blood and envelopes yang. It treats liver/kidney deficiency and weakness causing upward ascension which then gives rise to tinnitus and deafness. In addition, it treats vertigo and dizziness, low back and knee aching and feebleness, spermatorrhea, and night sweats.

3

Patent Medicines for Prevention in the Elderly

D ue to the physical condition of the elderly, they are more apt than others to suffer from cerebral vascular hemorrhagic disease, coronary heart disease, and other such conditions. This is because the elderly are constitutionally empty and weak due to advanced age and their resistance to disease is, therefore, weakened. Because of this, the elderly may easily catch any of the common diseases as well as the degenerative diseases mentioned above more typically associated with aging. The patent medicines described in this chapter treat the most common diseases associated with the elderly. Some of these medicines are supplements which support the righteous, while others are used to treat disease evils. Yet others both supplement and nourish and also eliminate disease evils.

I. Heart Pain

In Traditional Chinese Medicine, heart pain is subsumed under the traditional disease category of chest pain or *xiong tong*. The chest is the area where all the clear yang gathers and the chest qi (*zong qi*) is stored. When there is emptiness of yang qi, yin cold, phlegm fluids, blood stasis, and qi stagnation can all impede the flow of yang qi in the chest. It is said in Chinese medicine, "*Bu tong ze tong*." This means that if there is no free flow there will be pain. All of the above yin evils can contribute to heart or chest pain. In ancient texts this is called *zheng xin tong* or true heart pain, *jue xin tong* or inversion heart pain, *xin tong* or simply heart pain, and *xiong bi tong* or chest obstruction pain. These traditional Chinese disease categories are similar to angina pectoris associated with atherosclerotic heart disease but also include intercostal neuralgia. The main reasons for chest pain are as follows:

Qi Stagnation & Blood Stasis

Patients with this type of heart pain usually are easily depressed or angered and experience tightness and pain in their chest and ribs. If qi flow is not as smooth as it should be, the flow of blood will also not be as smooth as it should be. Thus qi stagnation leads to blood stasis, the vessels becomes stagnant and sluggish, and hence there is heart pain. The cause of most heart pain is extreme emotional overtaxation. The main signs and symptoms of qi and blood stagnation are a dull pain in the area of the chest and occasional fixed pain or palpitations with tightness in the chest. The tongue is dark in color with ecchymotic patches. The pulse is thready and astringent. For this type of heart pain with the symptoms mentioned above, the treatment principles should be to move the qi and activate the blood, free the *luo*, and stop the pain.

Yang Qi Insufficiency

Patients with this type of heart pain are prone to invasion by external cold thus causing stagnation of yin and cold. The resultant qi and blood stagnation will eventually become heart pain. This type of pain usually appears immediately after exposure to cold. The accompanying symptoms are shortness of breath and a stuffy sensation in the chest. In severe cases, pain may radiate to the back. The tongue has a thick, greasy, white coating and the pulse is slippery and wiry. The therapeutic principles for treating this type of heart pain is to free the yang, disperse cold, and stop pain.

Emptiness of Qi & Yin

Patients with this type of heart pain are empty of both their qi and yin and are constitutionally empty and weak. They will suffer from heart pain, shortness of breath, palpitations, spontaneous perspiration, dry mouth with scant saliva, a red tongue with scant coating, and a fine, weak, and forceless pulse with an irregular beat. The treatment principles for rectifying this imbalance are to boost the qi and nourish yin.

Yuan Qi Exhaustion

Patients who are extremely physically weak with exhaustion of their *yuan qi* often complain of such symptoms as heart pain, shortness of breath, great perspiration, incontinence of urine, and chilling of the four limbs and display facial pallor, fainting, a pale tongue with a white coating, and a minute, about to be exhausted, and possibly irregular pulse. The therapeutic principles for this type of heart pain are to boost the qi, rescue yang, and consolidate the desertion.

Phlegm Turbidity

Additionally, overeating greasy foods, overconsuming cold beverages, and drinking alcohol weaken and injure the stomach/spleen thus inhibiting their functions of transportation and transformation. The dampness which ensues may cause the arisal of phlegm, and phlegm turbidity may obstruct and cause stagnation of yang in the chest. This then results in heart pain,

73

tightness and a stuffy feeling in the chest, obesity, a thick, greasy tongue coating, and slippery, forceful pulse. The treatment principles for rectifying this condition are to aromatically perfuse the dampness and transform the turbidity, regulate the spleen, and transform phlegm.

Mao Dong Qing Pian ★♦

Ingredients: Radix Ilicis Pubescentis

Indications: Thromboangitis obliterans, arteritis, transient ischemic attacks, arteriosclerosis, and all types of heart disorders. Zhu says this medicine activates the blood, transforms stagnation, clears heat, and dissolves fire toxins. Because of this, Zhu says it is best prescribed for patients with either local or systemic signs of heat, such as swelling, redness, pain, warmth, thirst, constipation, a yellow tongue coating, and a rapid pulse.

Contraindications: Internal bleeding, such as bleeding ulcers, and hypermenorrhea and menorrhagia. This medicine can cause easy bruising in some patients.

Guan Xin Sou He Wan ★♦

Ingredients: Styrax, Lignum Santali Albi, Radix Saussureae Seu Vladmiriae, Borneolum, Olibanum, Cinnabaris. Zhu lists Semen Oroxyli Indici as an ingredient of this medicine and omits Saussurea.

Indications: Stuffy chest and heart pain due to coronary heart disease primarily due to phlegm turbidity and qi stagnation

Contraindications: Patients with cold stomachs should not use this medicine. Zhu says not to use this medicine if coronary heart disease is due mainly to blood stasis as characterized by fixed, stabbing pains possibly worse at night, a dark, purple tongue, and a deep, astringent pulse.

Dan Shen Sou Xin Pian ★
Dan Shen Pian ★

Ingredients: Radix Salviae Miltorrhizae

Indications: Coronary heart disease due to blood stagnation

Guan Xin Jing ★

Ingredients: Radix Panacis Ginseng, Radix Pseudoginseng, Radix Salviae Miltorrhizae, Lignum Dalbergiae Odorati, Styrax

Indications: Coronary heart disease, heart pain, and irregular heart beat

Mai Luo Tong ★

Ingredients: Not given

Indications: Coronary heart disease and stroke. This medicine frees the vessels and activates the *luo*, courses the qi and transforms stagnation, and relieves pain due to stagnation of qi and blood.

Ju Hua ★♦

Ingredients: Flos Chrysanthemi. This is not a patent medicine *per se* but merely the dried flowers of chrysanthemum which are frequently steeped in boiling water and drunk as a beverage tea by many older Chinese.

75

There are three types of chrysanthemum, white, yellow, and wild, and each has its own medicinal functions. Over the last 2,000 years, chrysanthemum has had may applications, such as calming the stomach and intestines, disinhibiting the circulation of blood, and relieving head wind. It has also been effectively used to treat headache, red eyes, and painful toxins.

According to modern research, chrysanthemum can also be used to lower blood pressure and enlarge the coronary arteries and is also antibiotic. For hypertensive as well as coronary heart disorder patients, white chrysanthemum is prescribed as a tea. It is used for lowering blood pressure and relieving dizziness and headache when taken with green tea. Yellow chrysanthemum can be used to relieve fever, red eyes, and sore throat due to an external hot disease. It has the power to clear heat, kill microbes, and clear inflammation.

Patients with heart pain and coronary heart disease can take 15 grams of white chrysanthemum infused in water twice per day. Drinking a combination of green tea and chrysanthemum is quite healthy for elderly patients, especially for those with hypertension.

Comparison of the Above Formulas

Mao Dong Qing Pian is primarily for the treatment of thrombo-angitis obliterans and arteritis due to blood stasis accompanied by heat and inflammation. Since it tends to work similar to blood thinners, it should not be used by persons with hemorrhagic disorders or those who bruise or bleed easily.

Guan Xin Sou He Wan primarily treats stuffy chest and heart pain due to obstruction by phlegm turbidity and qi stagnation.

It should not be used for heart pain due to emptiness of yin or yang or when there is empty fire. Nor should it be used in patients with more obvious stagnant blood.

Dan Shen Sou Xin Pian and *Dan Shen Pian* are for the treatment of heart pain and coronary heart disease due to blood Stasis.

Guan Xin Jing activates the blood and frees the vessels. It aromatically opens the orifices and stops pain. However, it also boosts the qi and consolidates the root. It is appropriate for treating coronary heart disease and heart pain characterized by heart qi insufficiency not maintaining normal control of the heart.

Mai Luo Tong activates the blood to relieve pain and courses the blood vessels. It moves the qi and disperses stagnation thus relieving stuffiness.

Ju Hua or chrysanthemum helps relieve heart pain and coronary heart disease especially in patients with hypertension and hypercholesteremia. In addition, it kills microbes and clears inflammation

II. Hypertension & High Cholesterol

Hypertensive patients typically complain of dizziness and headache. According to Traditional Chinese Medicine, hypertension is primarily caused by liver yang flaring upward and internal stirring of liver wind. Therefore, the treatment of hypertension in Chinese medicine is primarily based on levelling the liver and extinguishing wind. In order to accomplish this, there are several different methods.

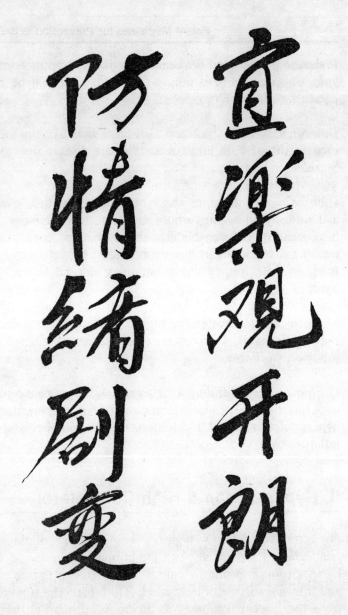

Be happy with a light, open view;
Guard against being seized by sudden
changes in emotion

For patients who are weak and suffer from exhaustion of liver/ kidney *jing* and blood thus giving rise to stirring of internal wind with dizziness, headache, tinnitus, restlessness, and weak low back and knees, medicinals should be used which supplement and boost the liver and kidneys, nourish yin and suppress yang, and therefore balance yin and yang.

Should the patient suffer from yang excess with a bad temper and is easily angered, this will cause transformative fire which will rise up and injure yin fluids. The resulting loss of balance between yin and yang with liver yang arrogantly ascending upward, will cause such symptoms as dizziness, headache, and distention of the head all of which are aggravated by anger, and a red face and cheeks, irritability, insomnia, excessive dreaming, a bitter taste in the mouth, a red tongue, dry stool, and dark yellow urine. For such patients, medicinals which boost yin and envelope yang, subdue the liver and extinguish wind should be used.

During extreme cases of liver/gallbladder fire flaring upward with dizziness, headache, red and painful eyes, swollen ears and deafness, painful ribs, a bitter taste in the mouth, irritability, a red tongue with a yellow coating, dry stool, and dark yellow urine, the treatment principles should be to clear and drain full liver/gallbladder fire, to put out fire and level yang.

1. Nourishing & Supplementing the Liver & Kidneys, Boosting Yin & Enveloping Yang

This pattern is due to deficiency and weakness of the liver and kidneys with emptiness of yin and arrogance of yang. Its main signs and symptoms are dizziness, headache, tinnitus, and weakness and feebleness of the lower limbs.

Jiang Ya Wan ★◆

Ingredients: Concha Margaritiferae, Radix Gentianae Scabrae, Radix Achyranthis Bidentatae, Flos Immaturus Sophorae Japonicae, Spica Prunellae, Radix Rehmanniae

Indications: Kidney yin insufficiency and upward ascension of liver fire with hypertension, headache, dizziness, tinnitus, and weakness and feebleness of the lower limbs

2. Levelling the Liver & Enveloping Yang

This pattern is due to arrogant ascension of liver yang with dizziness, irritability, a bitter taste in the mouth, and vexation.

Nao Li Jing ★

Ingredients: Raw Magnetitum, raw Hematitum, Rhizoma Pinelliae Ternatae, Borneolum, Concha Margaritiferae, Radix Achyranthis Bidentatae, fresh brewer's yeast

Indications: Dizziness, blurred vision, distention of the head and pain of the brain, insomnia, forgetfulness, and hypertension due to arrogant ascension of liver yang

Shu Xin Jiang Ya Pian ★

Ingredients: Radix Salviae Miltorrhizae, Flos Chrysanthemi, Radix Achyranthis Bidentatae, Radix Puerariae Lobatae, Ramus Loranthi Seu Visci, Semen Pruni Persicae, Semen Biotae Orientalis, Flos Immaturus Sophorae Japonicae, Flos Carthami, etc.

Indications: Hypertension with coronary heart disease. This formula relaxes the heart and lowers pressure as well as activates the blood and stops pain.

3. Clearing & Lowering Full Fire of the Liver/Gallbladder

This pattern is due to full liver/gallbladder fire flaring upward which manifests as dizziness, headache, a bitter taste in the mouth, red eyes, and other such conditions.

Long Dan Xie Gan Dan ★◆●

Ingredients: Radix Gentianae Scabrae, Semen Plantaginis, Radix Bupleuri Falcati, Fructus Gardeniae Jasminoidis, Radix Angelicae Sinensis, Radix Rehmanniae, Radix Glycyrrhizae, Radix Scutellariae Baicalensis, Rhizoma Alismatis, Caulis Akebiae Mutong

Indications: Dizziness, earache, tinnitus, pain in the ribs, a bitter taste in the mouth, a red tongue with yellow coating, and yellow urine caused by damp heat in the liver channel and itching in the genital area

Dang Gui Long Hui Wan ★

Ingredients: Radix Angelicae Sinensis, Radix Gentianae Scabrae, Herba Aloes, Fructus Gardeniae Jasminoidis, Rhizoma Coptidis, Cortex Phellodendri, Radix Scutellariae Baicalensis, Radix Et Rhizoma Rhei, Pulvis Indigonis, Radix Saussureae Seu Vladimiriae, Secretio Moschi Moschiferi

Indications: Full heat in the liver/gallbladder causing headache, red face, red, swollen, painful eyes, pain in the ribs, constipation, dark yellow urine, a wiry pulse, restlessness or spasm

Jiang Ya Wan ★◆

Ingredients: Semen Leonuri Heterophylli, Rhizoma Coptidis, Cornu Antelopis, Ramulus Uncariae Cum Uncis, Succinum, Radix Angelicae Sinensis, Lignum Aquilariae Agallochae, Radix Ligustici Wallichii, Rhizoma Gastrodiae Elatae, Radix Et Rhizoma Rhei, Radix Rehmanniae, Gelatinum Asini, Spica Prunellae, Cortex Radicis Moutan, Radix Achyranthis Bidentatae. This is the 20th Century formula manufactured by Beijing Tong Ren Tong. It is not the same as the *Jiang Ya Wan* described previously.

Indications: Vertigo and dizziness, pain and distention in the center of the chest, a red, flushed face, restlessness, a heavy sensation in the head, difficulty walking, and hypertension due to emptiness of yin and arrogance of yang. Zhu adds stiff neck, transient ischemic attacks, and temporary neurological symptoms such as facial or limb paralysis, diminished visual field, and abnormal sensations in the face and limbs.

Contraindications: Zhu cautions that this medication should not be used during pregnancy and that it should be used in full yang conditions only. He also suggests that its use be suspended temporarily during an external wind cold invasion and that this medicine may cause loose stools.

Jiang Ya Chong Ji ★

Ingredients: This powdered extract is composed of Caulis Clerodendri, Herba Apocyni Veneti, Radix Achyranthis Bidentatae, Flos Chrysanthemi Indici, Fructus Evodiae, Flos Immaturus Sophorae Japonicae

Indications: Hypertension

4. Lowering Cholesterol

The patent medicines described below are able to lower high cholesterol as well as lower high blood pressure and decrease fat. Thus they are good for obesity and hypertension.

Mai An Chong Ji ★

Ingredients: The ingredients of this powdered extract are not given.

Indications: Hypercholesterolemia and leukemia

Shan Zha ★♦

Ingredients: This is not a patent medicine *per se* but is simply Fructus Crataegi.

Indications: Hawthorne berries are good for relieving stagnant food, especially is due to overeating meat. They are also good for enteritis since they possess antimicrobial function and can stop diarrhea. In addition, hawthorne berries can lower high cholesterol and also relieve pain due to coronary heart disease. Elderly persons with high blood pressure, hypercholesterolemia, and coronary heart disease and heart pain can simmer 15 grams of hawthorne flakes and simmer in boiling water. Hawthorne flakes are made from hawthorne berries which have been boiled until soft, cut into slices, and dried for future use. The resulting liquid can be drunk as a medicinal tea over a long period of time.

III. Stroke & Paralysis

The major signs of stroke are sudden collapse, coma, aphasia, deviation of the mouth and wryness of the eyes, paralysis of the body, facial paralysis, or hemiplegia without coma. According to modern Western medicine, this includes cerebral vascular hemorrhage, cerebral infarction, cerebral thrombosis, cerebral angiospasm, subarachnoid bleeding, encephalitis, and facial paralysis. Since the attack comes suddenly and develops quickly, it is called in Chinese medicine wind stroke or sudden attack.

The causes of wind stroke are mainly due to emptiness of qi and blood in addition to worry, anger, improper diet, too much sex, or attack by external evils. Zhang Jing-yue of the Ming Dynasty said:

> Those who suffer from this disease usually do not take good care of themselves, are injured by extremes of the seven emotions, or indulge in sex and wine, all of which may harm the true yin of the five *zang* ... Initial emptiness of yin is followed by emptiness of yang. Yin is struck below and yang is exhausted above. This causes mutual loss of yin and yang and *jing* and qi do not communicate. This then results in sudden collapse and coma.

Therefore, to prevent wind stroke, one should focus on conserving one's life.

Wind stroke can be divided into two types: that which strikes the *jing luo* and that which strikes the *zang fu*. Due to their different nature, that which strikes the *jing luo* is less severe.

Because of constitutional emptiness, the *jing luo* become empty and the defensive qi is weak. Therefore, wind evil can easily attack the *jing luo* which then causes stagnation of the qi and blood. The circulation becomes sluggish and nutrients fail to nourish the *jin mai* or sinews and vessels. This may manifest as numbness of the hands and feet or sudden deviation of the face, stiffness of the tongue, uncontrollable salivation, or hemiplegia in severe cases. In such cases, it is necessary to dispel wind, free the connecting vessels, and nourish and activate the blood. If the patient has dizziness, headache, tinnitus, blurred vision,sore and weak low back and knees with sudden facial paralysis, stiffness of the tongue, difficult speech, hemiplegia, and a red tongue with a yellow coating, this condition is due to empty liver/kidney yin and internal stirring upward of empty yin fire. In this case, one should use medicinals to nourish yin and subdue yang, subdue the liver and extinguish wind.

Zang fu strike is a more severe condition. It manifests as sudden collapse and coma which may be of three different types: cold, hot, or yang qi collapse. If the patient suddenly collapses with a red face, coarse breathing, fever, bad breath, restlessness, gurgling sputum, jaws and fists tightly clenched, retention of feces and urine, and red lips and tongue with a greasy, yellow coating, and a wiry, slippery, and rapid pulse, this is yang *bi*. To treat this, one should clear heat and open the orifices, eliminate phlegm and extinguish wind. If the teeth are tightly shut, both hands are clenched, facial pallor, the sound of sputum in the throat, the four limbs lacking warmth, a white, greasy tongue coating, and a deep, slippery, slow pulse, this is yin *bi* and one must use spicy, warm medicinals to open the orifices, eliminate phlegm, and extinguish wind. If there is sudden collapse, coma, closed eyes by mouth agape, feeble breathing, cold limbs, profuse, cold sweating, incontinence of feces or urine, a minute pulse, and flaccidity of the tongue, this is yang qi collapse. For this, the treatment principles are to boost the qi, rescue yang, and secure the fallen.

Hemiplegia, difficult speech, aphasia, facial paralysis, and loss of memory are all side effects of wind stroke which require immediate attention and treatment with acupuncture, massage, and physical therapy. The treatment principles for the employ of these various modalities should be based on the individual patient's condition. For example, one might boost the qi and free the yang, activate the blood and free the *luo*, transforms phlegm and open the orifices, calm the liver and extinguish wind, or nourish and supplement kidney essence depending upon the needs of the presenting condition. In other words, there is no single, blanket treatment for stroke but each case must be diagnosed individually and treatment should be individually tailored based on a *bian zheng* or pattern discrimination diagnosis.

Su He Xiang Wan ★

Ingredients: Rhizoma Atractylodis Macrocephalae, Radix Saussureae Seu Vladimiriae, Cornu Rhinoceri, Rhizoma Cyperi Rotundi, Cinnabaris, Fructus Terminaliae Chebuale, Lignum Santali Albi, Benzoinum, Lignum Aquilariae Agallochae, Secretio Moschi Moschiferi, Flos Caryophylli, Borneol, Styrax, etc.

Indications: Wind stroke, loss of consciousness because of phlegm obstructing the orifices, heart pain due to coronary heart disease

Ren Shen Zai Zao Wan ★♦

Ingredients: Radix Panacis Ginseng, Radix Astragali Seu

Hedysari, Radix Conquita Rehmanniae, Radix Polygoni Multiflori, Plastrum Testudinis, Os Tigridis, Rhizoma Drynariae, Buthus Martensi, Lumbricus, Rhizoma Gastrodiae Elatae, Bombyx Batryticatus, Agkiistrodon, Ramus Loranthi Seu Visci, Rhizoma Dioscoreae Bixie Seu Hypoglaucae, Lignum Pini Nodi, Radix Clematidis Chinensis, Herba Ephedrae, Herba Cum Radice Asari, Herba Ledebourielliae Sesloidis, Rhizoma Et Radix Notopterygii, Radix Angelicae, Radix Puerariae Lobatae, Pericarpium Viridis Citri Reticulatae, Flos Caryophylli, Radix Scrophulariae Ningpoensis, Radix Et Rhizoma Rhei, Rhizoma Coptidis, Cinnabaris, Lignum Santali Albi, Rhizoma Curcumae Longae, Folium Agastachis Seu Pogostemi, Radix Rubra Paeoniae Lactiflorae, Radix Praeparatus Aconiti Carmichaeli, Cortex Cinnamomi, Radix Ligustici Wallichii, Lignum Aquilariae Agallochae, Radix Linderae Strychnifoliae, Rhizoma Cyperi Rotundi, Sanguis Draconis, Olibanum, Myrrha, Radix Pseudoginseng, Radix Angelicae Sinensis, Pericarpium Citri Erythrocarpae, Rhizoma Atractylodis Macrocephalae, Sclerotium Poriae Cocoris, Radix Glycyrrhizae, Semen Alpiniae Katsumadai, Massa Medica Fermentata, Calculus Bovis, Cornu Bubali, Concretio Silceae Bambusae, Borneolum, Secretio Moschi Moschiferi, Radix Saussureae Seu Vladimiriae, Rhizoma Praeparata Cum Fellem Arisaematis

Indications: Wind stroke, hemiplegia, spasms of the hands and feet, and unclear speech. Zhu adds that this medicine should be administered as soon as possible after the onset of stroke and that it can also be used preventively in patients who have already suffered transient ischemic attacks or other neurological problems associated with prestroke conditions.

Da Huo Luo Dan ★◆

Ingredients: Benzoinum, Borneolum, Radix Aconiti, Lignum

Aquilariae Agallochae, Radix Rubra Paeoniae Lactiflorae, Radix Cyathulae, Radix Ligustici Wallichii, Radix Et Rhizoma Rhei, Radix Angelicae Sinensis, Lumbricus, Flos Caryophylli, Semen Alpiniae Katsumadai, Herba Ledebouriellae Sesloidis, Sclerotium Poriae Cocoris, Radix Glycyrrhize, Radix Puerariae Lobatae, Rhizoma Drynariae, Radix Seu Herba Cum Radice Potentillae, Plastrum Testudinis, Radix Polygoni Multiflori, Os Tigridis, Rhizoma Coptidis, Radix Scutellariae Baicalensis, Folium Agastachis Seu Pogostemi, Bombyx Batryticatus, Herba Ephedrae, Myrrha, Radix Sausureae Seu Vladimiriae, Calculus Bovis, Agkistrodon, Radix Et Rhizoma Notopterygii, Pericarpium Viridis Citri Reticulatae, Radix Panacis Ginseng, Cortex Cinnamomi, Olibanum, Secretio Moschi Moschiferae, Radix Conquita Rhemanniae, Resina Praeparata Pini, Rhizoma Gastrodiae Elatae, Rhizoma Arisaematis, Radix Clematidis Chinensis, Zaocys Dhumnades, Radix Linderae Strychnifoliae, Cornu Rhinoceri, Herba Cum Radix Asari, Rhizoma Cyperi Rotundi, Radix Scrophulariae Ningpoensis, Sanguis Draconis

Indications: Wind stroke and paralysis, aching and soreness of the low back and legs, leg pain or stiff limbs. Naeser states that this medicine is used to treat the sequelae of both stroke and head injuries and should be commenced as soon as possible after the patient's condition has become stable. However, it should not be used for hemorrhagic conditions. Naeser also says that this medicine promotes the smooth circulation of qi and blood and relaxes the sinews. It expels wind and cold, stops spasm, and stops pain.

Xiao Shuan Tong Luo Pian ★

Ingredients: Not given

Indications: Cerebral hemorrhage causing neurological impairment, unclear speech, spasms and contractures of the hands and feet, contracture of the tongue, soreness and pain. The name, which translates as "Disperse the Plug Two Aged Ingredients", suggests that this formula is especially appropriate for phlegm blocking the orifices and the channels and connecting vessels.

Comparison of the Above Formulas

Su He Xiang Wan is a warm medicine which opens the orifices and treats apoplectic conditions associated with phlegm and cold. It is used as a first aid remedy to revive patients. For similar conditions associated with heat, *An Gong Niu Huang Wan* should be used instead.

Ren Shen Zai Zao Wan and *Da Huo Luo Dan* both supplement the qi and nourish the blood. They are used to treat the sequelae of strokes rather than the loss of consciousness itself. In addition, they activate the blood and free the *luo*. *Da Huo Luo Dan* can also be used to treat wind damp pain of the low back and legs.

IV. Cough & Asthma

Ke sou means cough. *Qi chuan* means wheezing and asthma. When wheezing and asthma are severe, patients may need to open their mouths to breath or raise their shoulders each time they inhale. Typically they cannot lie flat. Although cough and asthma are different symptoms, yet most of the time they occur together. Both are related to the lung channel and with other *zang fu* as well. The modern Western medical disease categories of bronchitis, pneumonia, bronchiectasis, bronchial asthma, emphysema, and tuberculosis, can all cause cough and wheezing. These are common diseases amongst the elderly. The causes of cough and asthma are as follows:

External Wind Cold Invasion of the Skin & Hair

The lungs are connected with the skin and hair. A wind cold invasion of the surface of the body obstructs and constricts the flow of qi through this layer of the body which is controlled by the lungs. This impairs the lungs' dispersing and descending function and may result in cough, tightness of the chest, a sore or itchy throat, cough with thin, white mucous, possible fever and fear of wind, head and body aches and pain, and a heavy sensation. The therapeutic principles for treating this type of cough and asthma are to disperse the cold, drain the lungs, stop the cough, and calm the asthma.

Wind Heat Invasion of the Lungs

Wind heat invading the lungs causes congestion of lung qi which results in cough or a stuffy feeling in the chest, cough with yellow mucous, thirst, sore throat, and fever with aversion to cold. The therapeutic principles for treating this type of cough and asthma are to disperse wind and clear heat, drain the lungs, stop the cough, and calm the asthma.

Phlegm Dampness

It is said in Chinese medicine that, "The spleen is the source of phlegm's arisal; the lungs are the place where phlegm is stored." This saying refers to the spleen's role in cough where there is more copious phlegm. If the spleen is empty, its transportation and transformation of water dampness will be impaired. It is also possible for evil dampness to invade the body externally. This dampness may give rise to phlegm. For cases where the phlegm is mostly white in color accompanied by fullness in the chest and abdomen, loss of appetite, fatigue, diarrhea, a thick, white tongue coating, and a slippery pulse, one should strengthen the spleen, dry dampness, transform the phlegm, stop the cough, and calm the asthma.

Emotional Aggravation

Longterm emotional aggravation and depression can stagnate the qi and injure the lungs. The lung qi loses its ability to drain and descend and coughing occurs. Sometimes qi stagnation transforms into fire, in which case liver fire assaults the lungs causing a dry cough with scant phlegm, chest pain, vexation and irritability, heart palpitations, and insomnia. In such cases, one must relax the liver and open stagnation, subdue the qi and calm the asthma, possibly clear and purge liver fire, moisten the lungs, and stop the cough.

Lung Qi Emptiness & Deficiency

If the lung qi becomes empty and deficient, this may cause cough, shortness of breath, a weak voice, aversion to wind and chill, a pale tongue and a deficient pulse. In such cases, the treatment principles are supplement and boost lung qi, stop the cough, and calm asthma. In cases where there is lung qi emptiness complicated by kidney qi emptiness, the patient has difficulty breathing in, emaciation, perspiration, chilled limbs, facial pallor, a pale tongue, and deep, weak pulse. In this case it is necessary to supplement the lungs and boost the kidneys, grasp the qi, and calm the asthma.

Emptiness of Lung & Kidney Yin

When there is chronic cough and asthma caused by emptiness

of lung yin or dual emptiness of lung and kidney yin, the symptoms seen will include dry cough or cough with blood, dry mouth and throat, afternoon fever, heat in the center of the hands and feet, restlessness, insomnia, a red tongue, and a fast, thready pulse. The treatment principles here are to nourish yin and boost the kidneys, moisten the lungs, and stop the cough.

1. Warming & Tranforming Cold phlegm, Stopping Cough & Calming Asthma

The patent medicines used for these purposes are warm and dry in nature. They disperse cold and relieve the surface. They warm and transform cold phlegm and stop cough and calm asthma.

Tong Xuan Li Fei Wan ★

Ingredients: Folium Perillae Frutescentis, Radix Scutellariae Baicalensis, Fructus Citri Seu Ponciri, Radix Glycyrrhizae, Pericarpium Citri Reticulatae, Radix Platycodi Grandiflori, Semen Pruni Armeniacae, Sclerotium Poriae Cocoris, Radix Peucedani, Rhizoma Pinelliae Ternatae, Herba Ephedrae

Indications: Cough due to wind cold with mostly white mucous, headache, stuffed nose, etc.

Fu Fang Chuan Bei Jing Pian ★♦

Ingredients: Herba Ephedrae, Radix Platycodi Grandiflori, Radix Polygalae Tenuifoliae, Radix Glycyrrhizae, Pericarpium Citri Reticulatae, treated Rhizoma Pinelliae Ternatae, Bulbus Fritillariae, Fructus Schizandrae Chinensis

Indications: Wind cold cough, asthma with profuse mucous which is difficult to expectorate, tightness in the chest, etc.

2. Clearing the Lungs & Transforming Phlegm, Stopping Cough & Calming Asthma

The patent medicines used in this category are good for clearing and purging lung heat, transforming phlegm, and stopping cough and asthma where there is yellow mucous, a dry mouth, thirst with a desire to drink cold liquids, and a red tongue with a yellow coating. These medicines can also be used for either chronic or acute bronchitis due to lung heat.

Qing Fei Yi Huo Hua Tan Wan ★

Ingredients: Radix Scutellariae Baicalensis, Fructus Gardeniae Jasminoidis, Bulbus Fritillariae, Cortex Phellodendri, Radix Platycodi Grandiflori, Radix Sophorae Flavescentis, Radix Peucedani, Radix Trichosanthis Kirlowii, Radix Et Rhizoma Rhei

Indications: Cough due to lung/stomach full heat with yellow mucous, constipation, dry mouth and tongue, sore throat, hematemesis, and hemoptysis

Qing Qi Hua Tan Wan ★◆●

Ingredients: Rhizoma Praeparata Cum Zingiberim Pinelliae, Rhizoma Praeparata Cum Fellem Arisaematis, Semen Trichosanthis Kirlowii, Semen Pruni Armeniacae, Fructus Immaturus Citri Seu Ponciri, Pericarpium Citri Erythrocarpae, Radix Scutellariae Baicalensis

Indications: Cough with difficult to expectorate, yellow mucous, a tight, full feeling in the chest, nausea and vomiting, a red tongue with a yellow, greasy coating, and a slippery, rapid pulse

Zhi Sou Ding Chuan Wan ★♦

Ingredients: Herba Ephedrae, Semen Pruni Armeniacae, Radix Glycyrrhizae, Gypsum

Indications: Pneumonia, acute bronchitis, fever, asthma, cough, thirst, a thin, white or yellow tongue coating, and a floating, slippery, rapid pulse

Qi Guan Yan Pian ★♦

Ingredients: Folium Eriobotryae, Fructus Zizyphi Jujubae, Radix Codonopsis Pilosuale, Folium Mori Albae, Radix Peucedani, Semen Pruni Armeniacae, Radix Polygalae Tenuifoliae, Pericarpium Citri Erythrocarpae, Bulbus Fritillariae, Flos Tussilagi Farfarae, Fructus Aristolochiae, Fructus Schizandrae Chinensis, Rhizoma Dessicata Zingiberis, Radix Platycodi Grandiflori, Radix Stemonae, Herba Cum Radice Asari, Herba Ephedrae, Cortex Cinnamomi, Sclerotium Poriae Cocoris, Pumice, Fructus Perillae Frutescentis, Radix Scutellariae Baicalensis, raw Gypsum, etc.

Indications: Bronchitis, cough with profuse phlegm, and phlegm asthma in the elderly

Ning Sou Wan ★

Ingredients: Bulbus Fritillariae, treated Rhizoma Pinelliae, Radix Platycodi Grandiflori, Fructus Perillae Frutescentis, Herba Dendrobii, Sclerotium Poriae Cocoris, Semen Pruni Armeniacae, Cortex Mori Albae, Pericarpium Citri Reticulatae, Fructus Germinatus Oryzae Sativae, Radix Praeparatus Glycyrrhizae

Indications: Cough and asthma due to lung heat with profuse phlegm

Zhi Ke Pi Pa Chong Ji ★

Ingredients: This granular extract is composed of Folium Eryobotryae, Radix Stemonae, Cortex Mori Albae, Radix Platycodi Grandiflori, Radix Et Rhizoma Cynanchi Stautoni

Indications: Wind injury (i.e., common cold), bronchitis, cough

Ke Chuan Pian ★♦

Ingredients: Herba Ephedrae, Gypsum, Fructus Schizandrae, Os Sepiae Seu Sepiellae, fried Semen Pruni Armeniacae, Radix Glycyrrhizae, Pumice

Indications: Asthma combined with bronchitis, asthma due to swollen bronchi, cough and asthma due to common cold

Ke Chuan Chong Ji ★

Ingredients: This granular extract is composed of Folium Isatidis, Radix Peucedani, Cortex Mori Albae, Rhizoma Pinelliae Ternatae, Radix Praeparatus Glycyrrhizae, Herba Ephedrae, Semen Gingkonis Bilobae, etc.

Indications: Asthma, cough, bronchitis, stuffy chest, difficult to expectorate mucous

Xiao Ke Chuan ★♦

Ingredients: Folium Rhododendri Daurici

Indications: Chronic and acute bronchitis, and cough due to common cold. Naeser says this medicine is good for treating cough due to common cold with copious mucous. She also says that this medicine is good for increasing the body's resistance to disease.

3. Nourishing & Boosting Lung Yin, Moistening Dryness & Stopping Cough

The patent medicines described below nourish lung yin and lung/kidney yin, moisten the lungs and stop cough. They are indicated for respiratory disease due to injury to yin, a dry cough with scant phlegm, tidal fever and night sweats, and possible hemoptysis in such diseases as pneumonia and chronic bronchitis.

Bai He Gu Jin Wan ★♦

Ingredients: Bulbus Lilii, Radix Angelicae Sinensis, Bulbus Fritillariae, Radix Glycyrrhizae, Radix Rehmanniae, Radix Conquita Rehmanniae, Tuber Ophiopogonis Japonicae, Radix Scrophulariae Ningpoensis, Radix Platycodi Grandiflori, Radix Alba Paeoniae Lactiflori

Indications: Tuberculosis, bronchitis, and inflammation of the throat due to lung kidney yin emptiness, sore dry throat, cough with bronchitis, mucous flecked with blood, hot vexation of the hands and feet, red tongue with scant coating, and a fine, rapid pulse

Li Gao ★

Ingredients: Tuber Ophiopogonis Japonicae, *Qiu Li* (identification unknown), Flos Tussilagi Farfarae, Bulbus Lilii, Bulbus Fritillariae, Rock Sugar

Indications: Cough due to empty yin, dry throat and mouth, hoarseness, spontaneous perspiration, and asthma

Mai Wei Di Huang Wan ★♦●

Ingredients: Radix Conquita Rehmanniae, Radix Dioscoreae Oppositae, Rhizoma Alismatis, Sclerotium Poriae Cocoris, Cortex Radicis Moutan, Tuber Ophiopogonis Japonicae, Fructus Schizandrae Chinensis, Fructus Corni Officinalis

Indications: Decline of both the lungs and kidneys, empty yin with internal heat causing cough and asthma, dry throat and mouth, redness of the cheeks, etc.

Li Fei Pian ★

Ingredients: Fructus Schizandrae Chinensis, Rhizoma Bletillae Striatae, Folium Eriobotryae, Concha Ostreae, Radix Stemonae, Cordyceps Sinensis, Bulbus Lilii, Gecko, Radix Glycyrrhizae

Indications: Tuberculosis, cough with blood flecked mucous, "thief perspiration" or night sweats due to empty heat, empty qi cough and asthma, chronic bronchitis, chronic cough, etc. Naeser notes that this medicine can be used for lung cancer if it conforms to an empty lung yin pattern.

Yang Yin Qing Fei Wan; also as a *Gao* or syrup & a *Tang Jiang* or liquid cough medicine ★♦

Ingredients: Radix Rehmanniae, Bulbus Fritillariae, Radix Scrophulariae Ningpoensis, Cortex Radicis Moutan, Tuber

Ophiopogonis Japonicae, Radix Glycyrrhizae, Herba Menthae, Radix Alba Paeoniae Lactiflorae

Indications: Tonsillitis, laryngitis, dry mouth and throat, throat swollen and painful, and rapid pulse. Naeser adds that this formula is used to treat dry cough or cough with little mucous and possibly some blood due to lung yin emptiness and empty heat.

3. Boosting the Qi & Supplementation of the Kidneys, Stopping Cough & Calming Asthma

These patent medicines supplement and boost the lungs and kidneys. They help grasp the qi and calm asthma. They are indicated for respiratory diseases in which there is constitutional emptiness, emptiness and weakness of the kidney qi, and inability for the kidneys to grasp the qi as in emphysema.

Ren Shen Bao Fei Wan ♦

Ingredients: Radix Panacis Ginseng, Bulbus Fritillariae, Semen Pruni Armeniacae, Radix Scrophulariae Ningpoensis, Fructus Schizandrae Chinensis, Pericarpium Papaveris Somniferi

Indications: Emptiness and deficiency of lung qi, deficiency and weakness of *jin ye* causing cough, cough and asthma, dry mouth and throat, and other such similar conditions.

V. Common Cold & Fever

Sudden changes in the weather, from cold to hot and *vice versa*, can easily cause attacks of the common cold (*gan mao*) and especially in the elderly due to their constitutional weakness and lack of strength of their *wai wei* or external defensive qi. Because common colds can cause or progress to more serious diseases if left untreated and again especially in elderly, it is important to treat such otherwise seemingly harmless diseases correctly, comprehensively, and speedily. Happily, there are a number of Chinese patent medicines which are quite effective for treating the common cold when administered based on a proper differential diagnosis.

According to Traditional Chinese Medicine, external evils attack the body by entering through the skin, mouth, and nose. Invasion of the skin (literally the *pi mao* or skin and hair) by wind cold evils obstructs the *wei yang* and then the qi and blood causing fear of cold, slight fever, headache, and body aches and pains. Because the lungs are connected with the skin and hair and because the nose is the orifice into which the lungs open, wind cold invasion of the skin and hair will also disrupt the function of the lungs and cause runny nose and sore throat. In addition to fear of cold, there may also be clear nasal discharge, hoarseness or laryngitis, and cough all due to lung qi not draining downward properly. In this case, fear of cold indicates a feeling of being afraid of cold not only when exposed to cold outside but also a fear of cold when inside the house. The treatment principles for treating the elderly who have been attacked by wind cold are to relieve the surface, disperse the cold, and boost their righteous qi.

Another kind of common cold is characterized by more pronounced or higher fever with only slight aversion to cold, more severe headache, dry throat and mouth, a swollen, painful throat, and cough. This is due to invasion by wind heat evil. In some cases, the disease may begin as a wind cold invasion and then the cold evil transforms into heat. In both instances, the treatment principle is to disperse wind heat.

1. Supplementation of Emptiness & Relieving the Surface

The following two patent medicines are both suitable for treating the common cold in persons with physical emptiness and weakness accompanied by and evidenced by spontaneous sweating due to emptiness.

Shen Su Li Fei Wan ★

Ingredients: Radix Panacis Ginseng, Folium Perillae Frutescentis, Radix Puerariae Lobatae, Radix Peucedani, Fructus Citri Seu Ponciri, Radix Platycodi Grandiflori, Rhizoma Praeparata Pinelliae, Sclerotium Poriae Cocoris, Radix Glycyrrhizae, Radix Saussureae Seu Vladimiriae, Rhizoma Recens Zingiberis, Fructus Zizyphi Jujubae

Indications: Constitutional emptiness weakness with attack of common cold, fatigue, fear of cold, fever, a stuffy sensation in the chest, hoarseness, cough with profuse phlegm, and a weak, forceless pulse

Yu Ping Feng Wan ★

Ingredients: Radix Astragali Seu Hedysari, Rhizoma Atractylodis Macrocephalae, Radix Ledebouriellae Sesloidis

Indications: Constitutional emptiness and common cold, lack of consolidation of the *wei* qi with fear of draft and spontaneous sweating, facial pallor, a pale tongue, and a floating, empty, soft pulse

2. Dispersing Cold & Relieving the Surface with Heavy Diaphoresis

The two patent medicines described below are both indicated for the treatment of wind cold *gan mao* accompanied by fear of cold, and edema of the limbs.

Gan Mao Qing Re Chong Ji ★♦

Ingredients: Herba Seu Flos Schizonepetae, Folium Perillae Frutescentis, Herba Menthae, Radix Platycodi Grandiflori, Semen Pruni Armeniacae, etc.

Indications: External invasion by wind cold, with aversion to cold, fever, whole body ache, headache, cough, stuffy nose, possibly a clear, runny nose, a bitter taste in the mouth, a dry throat and hoarseness, etc.

Huo Xiang Zheng Qi Wan ★♦●

Ingredients: Herba Agastachis Seu Pogostemi, Pericarpium Arecae, Sclerotium Poriae Cocoris, Radix Angelicae, Folium Perillae Frutescentis, Pericarpium Citri Reticulatae, Radix Platycodi Grandiflori, Rhizoma Atractylodis Macrocephalae, Cortex Magnoliae Officinalis, Rhizoma Praeparata Pinelliae, Radix Glycyrrhizae

Indications: Eexternal invasion of wind cold during the summer, internal injury due to cold dampness with fever and fear of cold, headache, fullness of the chest, chest and abdominal pain, nausea, vomiting, diarrhea, and thick, white, greasy tongue coating.

3. Clearing Heat, Dissolving Toxins, & Diaphoresis to Relieve the Surface

The following patent medicines are indicated for external invasion of wind heat and warm hot diseases, hot toxins, and fear of cold.

Yin Qiao Jie Du Pian ★♦●

Ingredients: Flos Lonicerae Japonicae, Fructus Forsythiae suspensae, Fructus Arctii Lappae, Radix platycodi Grandiflori, Herba Menthae, Rhizoma Phragmitis Communis, Radix Glycyrrhizae, Herba Lophatheri Gracilis, Herba Seu Flos Schizonepetae

Indications: Common cold due to heat and warm hot diseases during their early stage when heat has only penetrated the *wei fen*, fever, slight aversion to wind and cold, a swollen, painful throat, thirst, a red tongue with a white coating, and floating, fast pulse

Sang Ju Gan Mao Pian ★♦
Sang Ju Yin Pian ★♦

Ingredients: Folium Mori Albae, Flos Chrysanthemi, Herba Menthae, Semen Pruni Armeniacae, Radix Platycodi Grandiflori, Rhizoma Phragmitis Communis, Radix Glycyrrhizae, Fructus Forsythiae Suspensae

Indications: Common cold with fever, slight aversion to cold, cough and sore throat, headache, stuffy nose, but hot toxins not too great, and cough more obvious

Gan Mao Tui Re Chong Ji ★♦

Ingredients: This granular extract is composed of Folium Isatidis Daqingye, Radix Isatidis Seu Baphicanthi, Rhizoma Bistortae, and Fructus Forsythiae Suspensae.

Indications: Common cold with fever and more pronounced hot toxins, swollen, sore throat, laryngitis, tonsillitis, chronic and acute tracheitis

Jie Re Gan Mao Pian ★♦

Ingredients: Radix Isatidis Baphicanthi, Radix Scutellariae Baicalensis, Radix Puerariae Lobatae, Radix Scrophulariae Ningpoensis, Herba Cum Radice Violae Yedoensis, Herba Menthae

Indications: Internal heat with external cold accompanied by fever and chills, clear runny nose, the four limbs achy and tired, headache, cough, achy sore throat, and common cold with toxic condition

VI. Hot Diseases with Fever & Loss of Consciousness

Warm hot evils may attack the body from the outside through the nose and mouth and wind cold evil qi invading the skin and hair may transform into heat. Because the host qi of the body is yang and, therefore, warm, most diseases will likewise tend to be hot or transform into heat. Chinese medical theory calls this transformative heat in which case guest qi transforms into heat similar to the body's host qi. Chinese medicine divides warm hot diseases into four stages: *wei fen, qi fen, ying fen,* and *xue fen.*

When there is still aversion to cold, the heat is in the *wei fen* stage. The treatment principles at this stage are to relieve the surface and clear heat. A representative medicine for treating this stage of a *wen bing* or warm disease is *Yin Qiao Jie Du Pian.* However, if the exterior symptoms are no longer present and the evil heat has penetrated deeper, the signs and symptoms will be fever, thirst, heavy perspiration, a yellow tongue coating, and a big, forceful pulse. All these are indicative of the fact that heat has entered the *qi fen.* When evil heat penetrates even further to the *ying* and *xue* stages, there will be loss of consciousness, a purple tongue, a rapid pulse, high fever, spasms and convulsions, and epistaxis or hemoptysis. In such warm hot diseases, it is necessary to use cold medicinals which can dissolve heat such as the following.

An Gong Niu Huang Wan ★♦

Ingredients: Calculus Bovis, Cornu Rhinoceri, Secretio Moschi Moschiferi, Rhizoma Coptidis, Radix Scutellariae Baicalensis, Fructus Gardeniae Jasminoidis, Realgar, Borneolum, Tuber Curcumae, Cinnabaris, Margarita

Indications: Encephalitis, meningitis, toxin stroke (septicemia), urine toxins, toxin stroke associated with hepatitis, and wind stroke, delirium, irritability and vexation, spasm and convulsions, thirst, and constipation. Naeser says this medicine clears heat and dissolves fire toxin, opens the orifices of the Heart, and removes phlegm heat accumulation. It can be used in the treatment of stroke, seizures, and coma due to high fever in acute epidemic diseases. Naeser states that the pulse is rapid and full. In addition, this medicine can be used to treat hot evil attacking the pericardium and conditions similar to heatstroke.

Zi Xue Dan ★

Ingredients: Cornu Antelopis, Cornu Rhinoceri, Secretio Moschi Moschiferi, Cinnabaris, raw Gypsum, Glauberitum, Magnetitum, Radix Saussureae Seu Vladimiriae, Lignum Aquilariae Agallochae, Radix Scrophulariae Ningpoensis, Rhizoma Cimicifugae, Sodium Sulphate, etc. This list of ingredients differs from those given for a patent medicine of the same name by Naeser although both sources reference the *Tai Ping Hui Min Ji Ju Fang* as this formula's *locus classicus.*

Indications: Warm hot diseases with high fever, irritability and vexation, delirium, thirst, red urine, constipation, etc. Naeser says this medicine clears heat, opens the orifices, and dissolves fire toxins and is indicated for the treatment of encephalitis, meningitis, and other such hot diseases associated with coma, spasm, and convulsions.

Niu Huang Qing Xin Wan ★♦

Ingredients: Radix Angelicae Sinensis, Radix Ligustici Wallichii, Radix Glycyrrhizae, Radix Dioscoreae Oppositae, Radix Scutellariae Baicalensis, Radix Alba Paeoniae Lactiflorae, Tuber Ophiopogonis Japonicae, Rhizoma Atractylodis Macrocephalae, Massa Medica Fermentata, Pollen Typhae, Gelatinum Asini, Sclerotium Poriae Cocoris, Radix Panacis Ginseng, Radix Ledebouriellae Sesloidis, Rhizoma Dessicata Zingiberis, Radix Bupleuri Falcati, Cortex Cinnamomi, Radix Platycodi Grandiflori, Semen Germinatus Glycinis, Semen Pruni Armeniacae, Calculus Bovis, Secretio Moschi Moschiferi, Cornu Rhinoceri, Borneolum, Cinnabaris, Realgar, Cornu Antelopis

Indications: Spasm, stroke, paralysis, facial paralysis, coma, delirium, and dizziness due to heat entering the pericardium. It is used for the treatment of unconsciousness, delirious speech, uneasiness with high fever due to evil heat stiking the chest complicated by emptiness and phlegm.

VII. Swelling & Pain of the Throat & Mouth

Swelling and pain of the throat is typically related to fire and heat in the lungs and stomach. Stomach fire flaring upward can cause pain and swelling of the throat. Likewise fire heat scorching the lungs can injure the throat and cause hoarseness, swelling, and pain. In such cases, there will be dry mouth, a strong desire to drink, a red tongue with yellow coating, and dry stool. The therapeutic principles for treating this condition are to clear and purge lung/stomach fire and heat, dissolve toxins, and disinhibit the throat. If fire heat ascends upwards, it is necessary to free the stool. In addition, empty yin and flourishing fire can cause chronic swelling and pain in the throat. In this case, the treatment principles are to nourish yin and subdue fire.

Pain and swelling of the gums are also due to stomach fire flaring upward. For this the treatment principles are to clear and purge fire. The teeth are associated with the kidneys and that is why the elderly frequently have loose or painful teeth due to kidney deficiency and empty fire. For this, the therapeutic principles are to supplement the kidneys and subdue fire.

Ulceration of the mouth and tongue is mostly related to fire and heat in the two channels of the stomach and heart. Excess of stomach fire causes ulceration of the mouth, painful, swollen gums, and dry constipation. Flourishing heart fire primarily causes redness and pain of the tongue, red, burning urination, palpitations, and insomnia. In these cases, the therapeutic principles are to clear the stomach and subdue fire combined with clearing the heart and dissolving toxins.

Liu Shen Wan ★◆

Ingredients: Secretio Moschi Moschiferi, Calculus Bovis, Borneolum, Margarita, Venenum Bufonis, Realgar

Indications: Sore swollen throat, acute tonsillitis, boils, carbuncles, furuncles, diphtheria, and all kinds of abscesses

Hou Zheng Wan ★◆

Ingredients: Calculus Bovis, Venenum Bufonis, Realgar, Borneolum, Mirabilitum, Radix Isatidis Baphicanthi, Herba Lophatheri Gracilis, etc.

Indications: Red, swollen, hot, and painful throat, all kinds of throat inflammation, etc.

Qing Yin Wan ★◆

Ingredients: Radix Scrophulariae Ningpoensis, Radix Platycodi Grandiflori, Radix Sophorae Subprostratae, Fructus Sterculiae Scaphageriae, Herba Menthae, Borax, Radix Tinosporae, Rhizoma Belamcandae, Rhizoma Coptidis, Flos Lonicerae Japonicae, Tuber Ophiopogonis Japonicae, Fructus Terminaliae Chebulae, Radix Scutellariae Baicalensis, Fructus Gardeniae Jasminoidis, Bulbus Fritillariae, Radix Glycyrrhizae

Indications: Sore, swollen throat, hoarseness, and dry mouth and tongue due to lung/stomach heat

Niu Huang Jie Du Wan ★♦

Ingredients: Rhizoma Coptidis, Radix Platycodi Grandiflori, raw Gypsum, Cortex Phellodendri, Flos Lonicerae Japonicae, Fructus Viticis, Radix Angelicae, Radix Glycyrrhizae, Radix Ligustici Wallichii, Excrementum Bombycis Mori, Herba Menthae, Fructus Forsythiae Suspensae, Radix Et Rhizoma Rhei, Radix Ledebouriellae Sesloidis, Flos Inulae, Radix Scutellariae Baicalensis, Herba Seu Flos Schizonepetae, Fructus Gardeniae Jasminoidis, Flos Chrysanthemi, Calculus Bovis, Borneolum, Cinnabaris, Realgar

Indications: Ulceration of the mouth and nose due to accumulation of liver/lung/stomach heat, toothache, red, swollen, painful eyes, sore throat, red, swollen parotid glands, tinnitus and swollen, painful ears, head and eyes dizzy, constipation, and itchy skin

Niu Huang Shang Qing Wan ★♦

Ingredients: Rhizoma Coptidis, raw Gypsum, Radix Scutellariae Baicalensis, Herba Menthae, Plumula Nelumbinis nuciferae, Radix Angelicae, Radix Platycodi Grandiflori, Flos Chrysanthemi, Radix Ligustici Wallichii, Radix Rubra Paeoniae Lactiflorae, Radix Angelicae Sinensis, Cortex Phellodendri, Herba Seu Flos Schizonepetae, Fructus Gardeniae Jasminoidis, Radix Et Rhizoma Rhei, Radix Glycyrrhizae, Fructus Forsythiae Suspensae, Cinnabaris, Realgar, Calculus Bovis, Borneolum

Indications: Sore, swollen throat due to internal accumulation of heat, dry, ulceration of the mouth and tongue, swollen, painful gums, red eyes dues to wind and fire, and dry stool constipation

Bing Peng San ★

Ingredients: Borneolum, Borax, Cinnabaris, Mirabilitum

Indications: Swollen, sore throat, ulceration of the mouth and tongue, toothache and swollen, painful gums

Xi Gua Shuang ★♦

Ingredients: Fructus Citrulli, Saltpetre, Mirabilitum, Borneolum

Indications: Ulceration of the mouth and tongue, red, swollen throat, toothache and pain

VIII. Eye Diseases

The liver opens into the orifice of the eyes and it is blood which enables the function of sight. The liver and kidneys share a common source and *jing* and blood can mutually transform into one another. It can therefore be assumed that chronic, empty eye diseases are mostly due to liver/kidney *jing* and blood deficiency and weakness. Whereas, acute, red, swollen, and painful eyes are caused by full fire of the liver channel and arrogant ascension of liver yang.

Blurring of vision refers to failing to see things clearly. For example, when standing up all of a sudden after having been squatting for a while, the brain may feel all dark and there may be a ringing sound. As it is said, " Dizziness of all kinds in empty patients is due to emptiness of true water in the kidney channel." This is a common situation in the elderly as it is also in the weak patient. To treat this one needs to nourish yin blood, calm the liver, and clear the eyes.

When one loses one's eyesight and cannot see things clearly, this is called either night blindness or *qing mang* (clear-eyed blindness). Night blindness means that one cannot see clearly at night. *Qing mang* blindness is decreased visual acuity which is not influenced by the time of day. These are mainly due to emptiness of liver/kidney *jing*. If *jing* and blood are not sufficient, they fail to arise and nourish the eyes. Because decline of essence and blood are universal amongst the elderly, therefore decrease in eyesight and blurred vision are also relatively normal. However, if the elderly pay attention to conserving their life and protecting their *jing* and blood from exhaustion or use herbal medicines to supplement and nourish the liver/kidney *jing* and blood, these may retard the inevitable decrease in vision which typicaly goes along with aging.

Some elderly persons suffer from difficulty in opening and closing their eyes with weak eyesight or tiredness after staring at something. This is due to emptiness of both qi and blood. In such cases, one should boost the qi, nourish the blood, and increase one's constitutional vigor.

Sudden pain, burning, redness of the eyes with photophobia and tears, and difficulty opening the eyes is mostly due to liver fire flaring upward or wind heat in the liver channel. This is called *huo yan* or fire eyes or *chi yan* or red eyes in Chinese. In this case, it is necessary to clear and purge liver fire or disperse wind heat from the liver channel.

Shi Hu Ye Guang Wan ★♦

Ingredients: Herba Dendrobii, Radix Panacis Ginseng, Radix Dioscoreae Oppositae, Fructus Lycii Chinensis, Radix Glycyrrhizae, Fructus Schizandrae Chinensis, Tuber Asparagi Cochinensis, Fructus Citri Seu Ponciri, Sclerotium Poriae Cocoris, Rhizoma Coptidis, Radix Achyranthis Bidentatae, Flos Chrysanthemi, Radix Conquita Rehmanniae, Radix Rehmanniae, Radix Ligustici Wallichii, Semen Pruni Aremniacae, Semen Cuscutae, Radix Ledebouriellae Sesloidis, Cornu Antelopis, Cornu Rhinoceri, Tuber Ophiopogonis Japonicae, Semen Cassiae Torae, Herba Cistanchis, Fructus Tribuli Terrestris, Semen Celosiae

Indications: Liver/kidney dual deficiency, glaucoma, blurred vision, and internal eye obstruction

Qi Ju Di Huang Wan ★♦●

Ingredients: Radix Conquita Rehmanniae, Radix Dioscoreae Oppositae, Fructus Corni Officinalis, Sclerotium Poriae Cocoris, Cortex Radicis Moutan, Rhizoma Alismatis, Fructus Lycii Chinensis, Flos Chrysanthemi

Indications: Insufficiency of both the liver and kidneys with emptiness of yin and floating yang, blurred vision, sensitivity to light, tearing, dizziness, and tinnitus

Ming Mu Shang Qing Wan ★♦

Ingredients: Rhizoma Coptidis, Radix Platycodi Grandiflori, Radix Scrophulariae Ningpoensis, cooked Radix Et Rhizoma Rhei, Radix Scutellariae Baicalensis, Flos Chrysanthemi, Herba Menthae, Fructus Citri Seu Ponciri, Pericarpium Citri Reticulatae, Radix Glycyrrhizae, Radix Angelicae Sinensis, Radix Rubra Paeoniae Lactiflorae, Herba Seu Flos Schizonepetae, Fructus Fosythiae Suspensae, Fructus Tribuli Terrestris, Fructus Gardeniae Jasminoidis, Periostracum Cicadae, Radix Trichosanthis Kirlowii, raw Gypsum, Tuber Ophiopogonis Japonicae, Semen Plantaginis

Indications: Wind fire red eyes, eyes red, swollen, and painful, inflammation of the external eye, and other such acute eye diseases

IX. Headache

Headache is also a common problem amongst the elderly. There are basically two categories of headache in Traditional Chinese Medicine: 1) external attack and 2) internal injury. According to the *Nei Jing*, "If a person is empty of qi and blood, wind evil can attack the yang channels which go directly to the brain and thus cause headache."

Headache due to external invasion or attack is caused by wind, the beginning of one hundred diseases. As the sayings go, "When injured by wind, the top of the body will be attacked first," and "Only wind can reach the upper portions of the body." In everyday life, if we are not careful, wind may attack us. This external evil will attack our skin first entering the surface. Then it may go directly upward to the top of the head thus disturbing the clear yang and causing stagnation of the qi and blood. Therefore, headache occurs since pain is caused by stagnation. When wind cold attacks, cold constricts the *luo* and causes headache which radiates to the back of the upper back and neck. This pain is worsened when met with wind. Because of this, patients prefer to wear a hat or wrap up their head tightly. Such patients also complain of fear of wind and cold. In such cases, there is no particular thirst, a thin, white tongue coating, and the pulse is floating and tight. The therapeutic principles necessary for the treatment of such cases are to dispel wind, disperse cold, and stop the pain.

When wind heat attacks, people suffer from headache and dizziness or suffer from a hot, distended pain. If severe, one will have a severe headache which is worse when met with heat and which can be relieved by cold. Such patients also typically have a red face and eyes, thirst, restlessness, constipation, red urine, fever, aversion to wind, a yellow tongue coating, and a rapid pulse. In this case, the treatment methods should consist of dispelling wind, clearing heat, and stopping the pain.

When wind and dampness attack the clear yang and cause headache, the symptoms are headache which is like a tight band about the head which feels worse on rainy days, heaviness and tiredness of the four limbs, stuffy chest, sluggish digestion, difficulty urinating, loose stool, a white, greasy, turbid tongue coating, and soft, slow pulse. In this case, it is necessary to dispel wind, eliminate dampness, and stop the pain.

In chronic headache due to external attack or stagnation of phlegm fire, evil wind goes directly to the brain and turn into head wind headache. This type of headache comes and goes and recurs easily. It tends to recur when the weather turns bad and it also comes back when the patient is under emotional stress or is angry or depressed. At that time, the pain may be so severe that the patient cannot open their eyes or raise their head and their head may even feel numb.

Internal injury can also cause headache. As it is said, "The brain is the sea of marrow." This means that the brain is nourished by liver/kidney blood and *jing* and the essence of water and grains transformed and transported up to the brain by the stomach/spleen. Therefore, internal injury headache may be related to any of the three organs, the liver, kidneys, or spleen. The liver is related to the emotions and when a person is angry or depressed, liver yang may ascend to cause headache accompanied by dizziness. Such a headache is typically better or worse depending upon the patient's emotions. When the patient is angry, the headache is worse, the patient is not able to sleep well, and there will be ringing in the ears, a bitter taste in the mouth, a red tongue with thin, yellow coating, constipation, and red urine. In such cases, it is necessary to calm the liver, submerge yang, and clear and purge liver fire.

If liver/kidney *jing* and blood are deficient and weak, the sea of marrow will also be empty and the liver will not be nourished. empty yin and floating yang will, in this case, cause headache which is accompanied by an empty sensation, dizziness, weakness of the low back and knees, tinnitus, insomnia, and leukorrhea in women and premature ejaculation in men. The tongue will be red with scant coating and the pulse forceless and thready. The therapeutic principles for treating this type of headache are to nourish and supplement liver/kidney *jing* and blood.

If the qi is insufficient, the clear yang will not rise and the essence of water and grains will not ascend to nourish the brain. Such patients will suffer from a slight headache which is work after overexertion, shortness of breath, lethargy, palpitations, sluggish digestion, facial pallor, a pale tongue with coating, and pulse is empty, weak, and forceless. For this kind of complaint, one needs to boost the qi and ascend the yang. If headache is accompanied by a cold sensation in the head and cold limbs, a pale face, and a pale, flabby tongue, one should warm yang and supplement the kidneys.

If headache is due to assault above of phlegm turbidity and cold dampness, the symptoms will be headache, dizziness, nausea, vomiting of clear fluids, fullness in the chest and abdomen, a white, greasy tongue coating, and a wiry, slippery pulse. In this case, the treatment principles are to transform phlegm, harmonize the stomach, relax the liver, and lower rebellion.

When headache is caused by stagnant blood, the symptoms are chronic headache with fixed pain, sharp pain, a dark, purple tongue, and a thready, astringent pulse. For this type of headache it is necessary to activate the blood, transform stagnation, and stop the pain.

If headache comes after catching a cold or accompanies a *wen bing* or warm disease, hypertension, all kinds of brain diseases, neurosis, or neurasthenia, each of these must be treated differently according to the signs and symptoms and a discrimination of patterns of disharmony.

Chuan Xiong Cha Tiao San ★◆●

Ingredients: Herba Menthae, Radix Ledebouriellae Sesloidis, Radix Ligustici Wallichii, Radix Angelicae Duhuo, Herba Cum Radice Asari, Herba Seu Flos Schizonepetae, Radix Angelicae, Radix Glycyrrhizae

Indications: Headache due to external invasion of wind evil, frontal headache, headache at the vertex with fever, aversion to cold, stuffy nose, rhinitis, a thin, white tongue coating, and floating pulse. Although this medicine is called *san* or powder, it is available as pills and should be drunk with strong tea.

Xiong Ju Shang Qing Wan ★

Ingredients: Radix Scutellariae Baicalensis, Fructus Gardeniae Jasminoidis, Fructus Viticis, Rhizoma Coptidis, Herba Menthae, Flos Chrysanthemi, Fructus Forsythiae Suspensae, Herba Seu flos Schizonepetae, Radix Angelicae Duhuo, Radix Et

Rhizoma Ligustici Sinensis, Radix Platycodi, Radix Ledebouri ellae Sesloidis, Radix Glycyrrhizae, Radix Ligustici Wallichii, Radix Angelicae

Indications: Headache, dizziness, stuffy nose, tinnitus, toothache, and sore throat due to accumulation of lung/stomach heat and common cold due to wind evils

Qing Xuan Wan ★

Ingredients: Radix Ligustici Wallichii, Radix Angelicae, raw Gypsum, Herba Menthae, Herba Seu Flos Schizonepetae

Indications: External invasion of wind heat causing headache, headache, dizziness, and blurred vision due to heat in the liver channel, also headache due to hypertension and full fire ascending upwards

Comparison of the Above Formulas

Chuan Xiong Cha Tiao San disperses wind cold and stops headache. It is indicated for the treatment of headache due to external invasion of wind cold accompanied by fear of cold, fever, absence of perspiration, and other such symptoms.

Xiong Ju Shang Qing Wan and *Qing Xuan Wan* both dispel wind and clear heat. They are for headache due to external invasion of wind heat and heat in the liver channel. Both are indicated for the treatment of headache in a *tai yang* disease where there is dry mouth and parched tongue, vexation, dizziness, etc.

X. Diarrhea

Diarrhea may have several different causes among which are improper diet or inhibition of the stomach/spleen and intestines. Sudden onset of diarrhea with undigested food in the stool is typically the result of improper diet or contraction of cold. For this type of diarrhea, the treatment principles are to warm the middle and disperse cold, dry dampness, and stop the diarrhea. When diarrhea is accompanied by abdominal pain, burning in the anus, and/or vomiting, this is more typically due to heat and one must, therefore, clear heat, dry dampness, and stop the diarrhea.

If diarrhea is accompanied by blood, tenesmus, and abdominal pain with a feeling as if the organs have collapsed, a painful feeling of heat in the rectum, dark yellow urine, a dry mouth with a yellow tongue coating, and hot skin, these are all signs of attack by damp heat. The proper treatment of this consists of clearing heat, drying dampness, dissolving toxins, and stopping diarrhea.

In the elderly, the most common cause of diarrhea is emptiness and weakness of the spleen and kidneys in which case it is necessary to supplement and boost as much as possible within the limits of the situation.

Xiang Lian Wan ★

Ingredients: Rhizoma Coptidis and Radix Saussureae Seu Vladimiriae

Indications: Diarrhea due to damp heat, bloody diarrhea and tenesmus

XI. Constipation

Constipation in Traditional Chinese Medicine is not just a disorder of the large intestine but is related to spleen and kidney function as well. According to Chinese medicine, the six *fu* bowels desire to be free flowing at all times. The large intestine is a *fu* bowel and therefore it also desires to be free flowing. If it is not free flowing there will be constipation. Because of the relationships between the kidneys and spleen, the pre and postnatal roots, and the large intestine, healthy large intestine function is very important for the healthy functioning of the entire body. Likewise, ever since the Qing Dynasty, Chinese doctors have recognized the important reciprocal relationship between the large intestine and liver. Constipation tends to be associated with and aggravates many liver conditions in Chinese medicine and one way to treat such liver diseases is to assure the free flow of the large intestine. This is why constipation often accompanies such problems as heart disease, hypertension, and wind stroke. When patients with hypertension and lung and heart disease patients suffer from constipation, their symptoms are more severe. But when their bowels are open and free, their disease is less severe.

Constipation is a common problem amongst the elderly. Mostly, constipation in the elderly is associated with *jing* deficiency and scanty blood. Since blood and *jin ye* or body fluids share a common source, emptiness of blood can cause exhaustion of body fluids and fluid exhaustion of the large intestine is one of the causes of constipation. It is also possible for fire and heat to cause constipation by scorching the body fluids. Such fire and heat in the elderly are often the consequence of empty yin. Further, constipation in the elderly may also be due to emptiness of qi and decline of yang in which case yang qi is insufficient to transform and transport food. In such cases, there may be only one bowel movement per week or one in several days. When constipation is due to emptiness of yin and flaring of fire, one should nourish yin and subdue fire, moisten the bowels, and free the stool. When constipation is due to decline of yang, one must warm yang, boost the qi, and promote bowel movements. In some cases, constipation in the elderly may be due to accumulation of fire and heat in which case it is necessary to clear and purge fire and free the stool.

1. Moistening & Making the Stools More Slippery

The patent medicines described below all act to moisten the bowels and make the stools more slippery. They are indicated for the treatment of constipation in the elderly due to constitutional emptiness, deficiency of fluids, and parching of the blood.

Ma Zi Ren Wan ★◆●

Ingredients: Semen Cannabis Sativae, Semen Pruni Armeniacae, Radix Et Rhizoma Rhei, Fructus Immaturus Citri Seu Ponciri, Cortex Praeparatus Cum Zingiberim Magnoliae Officinalis, Radix Alba Paeoniae Lactiflorae

Indications: Dry heat of the stomach and intestines, constipation, and polyuria due to emptiness in the elderly

Wu Ren Wan ★

Ingredients: Semen Pruni Persicae, Semen Pruni Armeniacae, Semen Biotae Orientalis, Fructus Pini Tabulaeformis, Semen Pruni Japonicae, Pericarpium Citri Reticulatae

Indications: Constipation due to insufficiency of fluids in the

119

intestines and stomach

2. Clearing & Purging Full fire & Freeing the Stool

The following patent medicine are indicated for constipation due to liver/gallbladder full fire and flourishing of heart/liver fire with red eyes and bitter mouth, heart palpitations, and dry constipation.

Geng Yi Wan

Ingredients: Herba Aloes and Cinnabaris

Indications: Constipation due to flaring of heart/liver fire, heart palpitations, and insomnia

3. Tonification of Fire to Free the Stool

The patent medicine below is indicated to treat weakening of the *ming men* fire in the elderly and insufficiency of yang qi causing constipation.

Ban Liu Wan

Ingredients: Rhizoma Praeparatus Cum Zingiberim Pinelliae and Sulphur

Indications: Constipation in the elderly due to emptiness of yang

XII. Fullness & Distention of the Chest & Abdomen

Abdominal fullness without costal pain, fullness of the chest, and fullness of the stomach are all common in the elderly. When there is distention and the ribs are also painful, this is due to liver qi stagnation. The costal region is controlled by the liver. If anger causes rebellious counterflow of qi or emotional upset causes qi stagnation, this can cause fullness and distention with pain in the ribs. Sometimes such pain may occur on only one side. Stress and depression tend to aggravate this situation. These an also cause fullness and distention in the stomach or nausea and vomiting. This indicates that liver qi has invaded the stomach and that there is disharmony between the liver and stomach. Or there can be loss of appetite, lose stools, and abdominal pain due to liver qi invading the spleen with resultant disharmony of the liver and spleen. In such cases, one should either harmonize the liver and stomach or harmonize the liver and spleen as indicated.

Chest fullness manifests as fullness in the chest, difficulty breathing, and sighing. Some people may feel like there is qi residing in their diaphragm which refuses to descend. They feel relieved when qi does go down, i.e., they pass gas. If this is the case and there is abdominal fullness and distention plus constipation, this usually means there is stagnation of both qi, dampness, and food. For this condition, the treatment principles are to move the qi, eliminate dampness, and clear the intestines. Sometimes emptiness of qi causes fullness of the diaphragm with shortness of breath and such general emptiness signs and symptoms as fatigue, feeble voice, and loss of breath on slight exertion. For this, one needs to supplement the qi and must not use medicinals to move the qi or eliminate dampness.

The stomach is in the upper abdomen. When the stomach feels full and there is discomfort and distention this may be differentiated into empty and full categories. The full type is caused by stagnation of qi, dampness disturbing the stomach/spleen, and overeating causing food stagnation in the stomach. The symptoms of this are a thick, greasy tongue coating and bad breath. In this case, the therapeutic principles are to move the qi and disperse distention, dry the dampness and harmonize the middle, and disperse food stagnation. However, in the elderly stomach distention and fullness is mostly due to spleen emptiness with weakened transportation and transformation. This is called empty distention and is characterized by a small appetite with fullness after eating. In this case, one should strengthen the spleen and boost the stomach, move the qi and disperse the distention.

Lower abdominal fullness and distention may have either of two causes. The first is constipation. Many older people only have one bowel movement every couple of days. Therefore their lower abdomen will be full. In this case, one should moisten the intestines and move the stools in order to disperse the digestate. Some older persons feel as if their qi stays in their lower abdomen. This tends to feel worse at night. This also is a species of empty distention. It is a sign of stomach/spleen emptiness. In this case, it is necessary to strengthen the spleen and move the qi to disperse stagnation.

Abdominal and chest fullness and distention are very commonly encountered in clinical practice. Therefore, there are lots of Chinese patent medicines to treat these conditions.

1. Relaxing the Liver, Activating the Qi, Harmonizing the Stomach, & Stopping Pain

The two patent medicines described below soothe the liver, regulate the qi, harmonize the stomach, and stop pain. They are indicated for liver depression and qi stagnation, liver qi invading the stomach/spleen, distention and pain in the abdomen and chest, indigestion, and other similar conditions.

Shu Gan Wan ★♦

Ingredients: Lignum Aquilariae Agallochae, Semen Myrsticae Fragrantis, Fructus Seu Semen Amomi, Rhizoma Cyperi Rotundi, Tuber Corydalis Yanhusuo, Cortex Magnoliae Officinalis, Fructus Meliae Toosendanis, Rhizoma Curcumae Longae, Radix Saussureae Seu Vladimiriae, Radix Alba Paeoniae Lactiflorae, Sclerotium Poriae Cocoris, Fructus Citri Seu Ponciri, Pericarpium Citri Reticulatae, Fructus Amomi Cardamomi

Indications: Pain in the flanks due to liver qi stagnation and/or disharmony of the liver and stomach, stomach discomfort, indigestion, belching, and loss of appetite

Chen Xiang Hua Qi Wan ★♦

Ingredients: Lignum Aquilariae Agallochae, Radix Glycyrrhizae, Radix Saussureae Seu Vladimiriae, Pericarpium Citri Reticulatae, Fructus Seu Semen Amomi, Massa Medica Fermentata, Rhizoma Cyperi Rotundi, Herba Agastachis Seu Pogostemi, etc.

Indications: Fullness of the chest and abdomen due to liver/stomach qi stagnation, belching, lack of appetite, etc.

123

Comparison of the Above Formulas

Shu Gan Wan soothes the liver and harmonizes the stomach and is indicated for liver depression and qi stagnation and disharmony of the liver and stomach. Besides stopping pain, these pills balance and harmonize the spleen and stomach and disperse stagnant food.

Chen Xiang Hua Qi Wan balance and harmonize the spleen and stomach and invigorate the spleen to improve digestion. They are indicated for lack of harmony between the liver and stomach and food stagnation with fullness and distention of the stomach and abdomen.

2. Moving the Qi, Leading Away Stagnation, & Freeing the Stomach and Intestines

The two patent medicines described below are intended to move the qi, lead away stagnation, and promote free bowel movements. They are indicated for the treatment of qi stagnation and stagnant food, accumulation of dampness in the stomach/spleen, distention and pain, and bowel movements which are not free flowing. Unfortunately only two of the six Chinese patent medicines described in this section of the root text are available currently in the United States.

Mu Xiang Shun Qi Wan ★◆

Ingredients: Radix Saussureae Seu Vladimiriae, Fructus Immaturus Citri Seu Ponciri, Pericarpium Citri Reticulatae, Rhizoma Cyperi Rotundi, Semen Arecae, Rhizoma Atractylodis, Fructus Seu Semen Amomi, Cortex Magnoliae Officinalis, Radix Glycyrrhizae, Pericarpium Viridis Citri Reticulatae

Indications: Chest and abdominal distention and stuffiness due to qi stagnation not soothed

Yue Ju Wan ♦

Ingredients: Rhizoma Atractylodis, Rhizoma Cyperi Rotundi, Radix Ligustici Wallichii, Massa Medica Fermentata, Fructus Gardeniae Jasminoidis

Indications: Fullness, distention, and pain of the chest and abdomen due to stagnation of qi, blood, phlegm, fire, dampness, and food, belching and vomiting with undigested food, etc.

Comparison of the Above Formulas

Mu Xiang Shun Qi Wan primarily moves the qi and treats chest and abdominal distention due to the qi not being soothed and free flowing.

Yue Ju Wan, on the other hand, disperses combined stagnation of dampness, qi, food, and fire and treats chest and abdominal distention and stuffiness and loss of appetite due to interdependent and combined presence of these.

3. Drying Dampness & Moving the Qi, Dispersing Distention & Relieving Fullness

The patent medicines described below dry dampness, move the qi, balance and regulate the stomach/spleen, disperse distention, and relieve fullness. They are indicated for the treatment of accumulation of dampness and stuffing of qi causing distention and fullness, food stagnation, vomiting, diarrhea, and a greasy, turbid tongue coating.

Ping Wei Wan ★♦
Xiang Sha Ping Wei Wan ★♦

Ingredients: *Ping Wei Wan* is composed of Rhizoma Atractylodis, Pericarpium Citri Reticulatae, Cortex Magnoliae Officinalis, and Radix Glycyrrhizae. *Xiang Sha Ping Wei Wan* is composed of the same ingredients plus Radix Saussureae Seu Vladimiriae and Fructus Seu Semen Amomi.

Indications: *Ping Wei Wan* treats accumulation of dampness and turbidity accumulating in the middle and lack of harmony between the spleen and stomach, loss of taste for food, stuffy chest and abdominal distention, belching and vomiting, fatigue, diarrhea, and a greasy, turbid tongue coating. *Xiang Sha Ping Wei Wan* additionally calms and disperses the stomach. It moves the qi, restores the appetite, and promotes digestion.

Xiang Sha Yang Wei Wan ★♦

Ingredients: Rhizoma Atractylodis Macrocephalae, Pericarpium Citri Reticulatae, Sclerotium Poriae Cocoris, Rhizoma Praeparata Pinelliae, Fructus Seu Semen Amomi, Rhizoma Cyperi Rotundi, Radix Saussureae Seu Vladimiriae, Fructus Immaturus Citri Seu Ponciri, Semen Alpiniae Katsumadai, Herba Agastachis Seu Pogostemi, Cortex Magnoliae Officinalis, Radix Glycyrrhizae, Fructus Zizyphi Jujubae, Rhizoma Recens Zingiberis

Indications: Accumulation of dampness and stuffing of qi, lack of appetite, abdominal distention and stuffiness, vomiting of sour water, fatigue of the four limbs

Comparison of the Above Formulas

Ping Wei Wan transforms dampness and turbidity and is, therefore, indicated for accumulation and stuffing of dampness and turbidity in the middle burner/stomach/spleen accompanied by lack of appetite, abdominal distention and fullness, possible vomiting and/or diarrhea, and a greasy, turbid tongue coating. *Xiang Sha Ping Wei Wan* additionally restores the appetite (literally opens the stomach), moves the qi, and relieves distention.

Xiang Sha Yang Wei Wan transforms dampness and turbidity, moves qi stuffiness, and wakes the spleen. It is indicated for the treatment of accumulation of dampness, stuffing of the qi, and inhibition of spleen transportation and transformation, accompanied by loss of appetite, fullness and distention of the abdomen, etc.

4. Eliminating & Leading Away Food Accumulation & Stagnation

The patent medicine below is indicated for improving the digestive function of the stomach and intestines when too much food has been eaten. It calms the stomach/spleen and improves digestion when there is accumulation and stagnation not descending, with fullness and distention.

Bao He Wan ★♦

Ingredients: Fructus Crataegi, Massa Medica Fermentata, Rhizoma Praeparata Pinelliae, Sclerotium Poriae Cocoris, Pericarpium Citri Reticulatae, Fructus Forsythiae Suspensae, Semen Raphani Sativi

127

Indications: Food stagnation causing fullness and distention of the chest and abdomen, acid regurgitation, loss of appetite, and constipation or diarrhea

5. Moving the Qi & Dispersing Cold to Treat *Shan Qi*

The following patent medicine moves the qi and stops pain, disperses cold and tonifies fire, soothes the liver, and transforms stagnation in the treatment of *shan qi* or problems in the inguinal region such as hernia.

Hui Xiang Ju He Wan ★

Ingredients: Semen Citri, Cortex Magnoliae Officinalis, Semen Pruni Persicae, Thallus Laminariae, Caulis Akebiae Mutong, Cortex Cinnamomi, Fructus Meliae Toosendan, Rhizoma Corydalis Yanhusuo, Sargassum, Radix Saussureae Seu Vladmiriae, Fructus Immaturus Citri Seu Ponciri, Fructus Foeniculi Vulgaris, Thallus Algae

Indications: *Shan qi*, hernia and swollen scrotum, pain and distention of the inguinal region

XIII. Loss of Normalcy of Urination & Edema

Loss of normalcy of urination implies frequency of urination, post urination dribbling, difficulty urinating, turbid urine, painful urination, and blood in the urine with edema and other similar conditions. It is mostly related to loss of normalcy of the bladder and kidney function.

The bladder is the water *fu* which stores urine. The kidneys are the water *zang*. It is the kidney's *ming men* fire which controls the *qi hua* transformation of water. The opening and closing of the gate of the bladder is also related to the normal secretion of urine. Because the kidneys gradually become empty in the elderly and their *ming men* fire is weakening, this decreases the opening and closing function of the bladder. Therefore, the bladder loses its ability to urinate and loses its control of the opening and closing of the gate of water. This, in turn, leads to frequent urination, incontinence, urinary dribbling, and difficult urination. Thus the bladder becomes full and dysfunctional or the prostate gland becomes enlarged. In such cases, it is necessary to warm the kidneys and control the urination, supplement the kidneys, and supplement yang to improve bladder function. Edema is also related to the spleen's function of transporting and transforming water and the lungs' function of dispersing the water passageways or *shui dao*. Therefore, in addition, it is also always appropriate to strengthen the spleen

and disinhibit water and to disperse the lungs in order to move water.

Painful and difficult urination are categorized as *lin zheng* in Chinese medicine. *Lin* is mostly due to damp heat in the bladder. As it is said,

> When the kidneys are empty, urination is
> frequent;
> When the bladder is hot, urination is difficult;
> Frequent and difficult urination are called *lin*.

When the urine is colored mostly yellow with distention of the lower abdomen, and low back pain, the treatment principles are to clear heat, disinhibit dampness, disinhibit urination, and free *lin* or strangury.

Dripping, painful urination with blood in the urine is called *xue lin* or blood *lin*. In this case it is necessary to clear heat, cool the blood, and to stop bleeding in the initial, acute stage. In chronic cases which recur after stress or hard work, one should nourish yin, boost the qi, cool the blood, and stop bleeding.

Difficult urination with crystal clear urine is called either *sha* or sandy *lin* or *shi* or stone *lin*. The signs and symptoms here are due to urinary stones and for this one should disinhibit the urine, transform the stones, and free the strangury.

When the urine is turbid but without pain, this called *gao lin* or fat *lin*. This is due to damp heat or cold dampness pouring downward. In this case, the treatment principles are to clear and disinhibit dampness and heat or to boost the qi, raise yang, and separate clear from turbid.

1. Disinhibiting Water & Dispersing Swelling

The six patent medicines described in this section of the main text all disinhibit urination and disperse swelling. They treat edema, stagnation of water in the chest and abdomen, and internal accumulation of phlegm. Unfortunately, none of these patent medicines are currently available in the United States. However, one of these formulas is available as desiccated extract from the companies which supply *Kanpo Yaku* medicinals, such as Qualiherbs, and Brion.

Wu Ling San ●

Ingredients: Sclerotium Poriae Cocoris, Rhizoma Alismatis, Sclerotium Polypori Umbellati, Cortex Cinnamomi, Rhizoma Atractylodis Macrocephalae

Indications: External or surface condition with internal stagnation of water which is not moving and which causes headache, fever, difficulty urinating, edema, diarrhea, and vomiting after drinking water

2. Disinhibiting Urination, Freeing *Lin* & Dispelling Stones

Some of the patent medicines described in this section of the main text disinhibit urination, free *lin* or urinary strangury, clear heat, and dissolve toxins. Others disinhibit urination and kill microbes. And yet others eliminate stagnation due to stones and stop bleeding. In general, they are used to treat cystitis, urethritis, nephrolithiasis, and other such conditions. Three of five of the patents described in the main text are available in the United States.

Bei Xie Feng Qing Wan ★

Ingredients: Rhizoma Dioscoreae Bixie Seu Hypoglaucae, Radix Lindera Strychnifoliae, Rhizoma Acori Graminei, Fructus Alpiniae Oxyphyllae, Radix Glycyrrhizae

Indications: Empty cold and cold dampness in the bladder with polyuria, turbid urine, dribbling and pain

Pai Shi Chong Ji ★

Ingredients: Herba Jinqiancao, Semen Plantaginis, Folium Pyrrosiae, Ramus Lonicerae Japonicae, etc.

Indications: Stones in the kidney, ureters, and bladder

Shi Lin Tong ★

Ingredients: Herba Jinqiancao

Indications: All types of stones in the urinary system

3. Assist Yang & Control Urination

The single patent medicine described below is used to warm kidney yang in cases of polyuria, incontinence, and dribbling due to kidney emptiness.

Sang Piao Xiao San ●

Ingredients: Ootheca Mantidis, Os Draconis, Radix Panacis Gineng, Rhizoma Acori Graminei, Sclerotium Pararadicis Poriae Cocoris, Radix Polygalae Tenuifoliae, Radix Angelicae, Plastrum Testudinis

Indications: Dual heart/kidney emptiness with polyuria and incontinence, forgetfulness or absentmindedness, a white tongue coating, and a fine, weak pulse

XIV. Wind Damp Obstruction & Pain

Bi means obstruction or a blockage through which there is no free flow. If wind, cold, and/or damp evils attack the body they may cause sluggish movement of the qi and blood and stagnation and accumulation in the channels and connecting vessels. This inhibits the movement and function of the joints, the sinews and bones, and the muscles causing soreness and pain, heaviness, numbness, and swelling of the joints. All these conditions are categorized as wind damp *bi* pain and are called wind damp joint pain. There are several different causes of wind damp *bi* pain:

Weak Constitution & Emptiness of Defensive Yang

An empty, weak constitution with a weak *wai wei* or external defence may allow the body to attacked by wind, cold, and damp evils. As it is said, "When evil qi attacks, there is emptiness of qi," and, "When the constitution is empty, there is lack of ability to defend, and wind, cold, and damp evils will cause *bi*." This means that wind, cold, and dampness can attack the body when the body itself is empty and weak. Therefore, supporting the Righteous qi is the main principle for preventing wind damp pain.

Exposure to External Cold & Dampness

Even if the body is not weak, if one lives in a cold, damp place for a long time or lives where hot and cold weather alternate repeatedly, or if one walks through the water or in the rain, due to these causes cold, damp evils may disturb the flow of qi and blood thus giving rise to *bi* and pain due to stagnation. Therefore, one should be aware not to live in a cold, damp place.

Depending upon the different types of wind/cold/damp *bi*, there are varying signs and symptoms.

Pain which migrates from joint to joint with difficulty moving the joint or aversion to wind and cold is wind cold *bi*. The nature of wind is movement and so wind *bi* is characterized by wandering or migrating pain. In such cases, the therapeutic principles are to dispel wind, free the connecting vessels, disperse the cold, and stop the pain.

Joint pain which is severe, fixed, with difficult movement, and which is worse with cold but relieved by heat, is not red, and is without heat in the joints is due to cold. Cold causes stagnation and so the pain is both fixed and severe. Because cold is also contracting in nature, there is difficulty moving the joints. In this case, it is necessary to disperse cold, stop pain, dispel wind, and free the collaterals. This is the reverse emphasis compared to predominantly wind or wandering *bi*.

When a joint is painful or swollen and distended with heaviness of the arms and legs, difficult movement, fixed pain or numbness of the skin, these are signs and symptoms of predominating dampness. dampness's nature is to percolate downward and to be heavy. Therefore, the body feels heavy, there is difficulty moving, and fixed pain with numbness. The therapeutic principles for treating this type of damp *bi* are to eliminate dampness and disperse cold, dispel wind and free the *luo*.

If the joints is red, swollen, hot, and painful with pain so severe as to be unbearable but migrating and relieved by cold, difficulty moving, fever, aversion to cold, sweating, thirst, and irritability, these are all signs of severe heat. In order to treat this kind of inflammation of the joints, it is necessary to clear heat and purge fire, dispel wind and free the connecting vessels.

1. Supplementing, Boosting, & Strengthening; Relieving Wind Dampness; & Freeing the Channels & Connecting Vessels

The patent medicines described below all are composed of supplementing and boosting medicinals which support the righteous and consolidate the root. In addition, they relieve wind dampness and free the channels and connecting vessels, disperse cold and stop pain for the treatment of wind, damp, and cold evils causing *bi* obstruction in a person with inability to recover and injury of their righteous qi. They are also indicated for persons who are constitutionally empty and weak and suffering from wind/cold/damp evils and for persons suffering from low back and knee pain due to kidney emptiness, lack of strength of the legs, and similar conditions.

Hu Gu Jiu ★

Ingredients: This medicinal wine is composed of Os Tigridis, Rhizoma Dioscoreae Bixie Seu Hypoglaucae, Radix Achyranthis Bidentatae, Radix Conquita Rehmanniae, Pericarpium Citri Reticulatae, Rhizoma Polygonati, Radix Angelicae Sinensis, Radix Angelicae Duhuo, Radix Linderae Strychnifoliae, Cortex Radicis Acanthopanacis, Rhizoma Atractylodis, Radix Ledebouriellae Sesloidis, Pericarpium Viridis Citri Reticulatae, Cortex Radicis Moutan, Radix Ligustici Wallichii, Radix Angelicae, Fructus Chaenomelis Lagenariae, Radix Alba Paeoniae Lactiflorae, Radix Lithopsermi Seu Arnebiae, Fructus Lycii Chinensis, Flos Carthami, Fructus Psoraleae Corylifoliae, Radix Aconiti Chuanwu, Radix Aconiti Kusnezoffii Seu Caowu, Radix Saussureae Seu Vladimiriae, Flos Caryophylli, Fructus Citri Sacrodactylis, Fructus Seu Semen Amomi, Radix Panacis Ginseng, Cornu Cervi Parvum, Cortex Eucommiae Ulmoidis, Cortex Cinnamomi, Olibanum, Myrrha, Lignum Pini Nodi, Lignum Santali Albi, Radix Et Rhizoma Notopterygii, Semen Coicis Lachryma-jobi, Herba Epimedii, Secretio Moschi Moschiferi. Although both the main text and Zhu say the versions of *Hu Gu Jiu* they describe are made by Beijing Tong Ren Tong, there is some discrepancy in the identification of ingredients and at least one is definitely misidentified by Zhu.

135

Indications: Wind damp joint pain, tingling and numbness of the four limbs, low back and leg soreness and pain, etc.

Tian Ma Wan ★♦

Ingredients: Rhizoma Gastrodiae Elatae, Radix Achyranthis Bidentatae, Radix Scrophulariae Ningpoensis, Rhizoma Dioscoreae Bixie Seu Hypoglaucae, Cortex Eucommiae Ulmoidis, Radix Et Rhizoma Notopterygii, Radix Rehmanniae, Radix Angelicae Duhuo, Radix Praeparatus Aconiti Carmichaeli

Indications: Wind damp *bi* and pain, tingling and numbness of the hands and feet, and difficulty walking

Guo Gong Jiu ★

Ingredients: This medicinal wine is composed of Radix Angelicae Sinensis, Os Tigridis, Radix Angelicae Duhuo, Carapax Amydae, Rhizoma Dioscoreae Bixie Seu Hypoglaucae, Radix Ledebouriellae Sesloidis, Radix Gentianae Macrophyllae, Radix Achyranthis Bidentatae, Lignum Pini Nodi, Excrementum Bombycis Mori, Fructus Lycii Chinensis, *Jia* or *Qie Geng* (identification unknown), grain alcohol

Indications: Numbness and tingling of the four extremities, wind damp *bi* and pain, inhibition of the joints, discomfort of the hands and feet

Hu Gu Mu Gua Wan ★

Ingredients: Os Tigridis, Radix Angelicae, Radix Ligustici Wallichii, Caulis Piperis, Radix Aconiti Caowu, Radix Clemetidis Chinensis, Fructus Chaenomelis Lagenariae, Radix Aconiti Chuanwu, Radix Angelicae Sinensis, Rhizoma Sinomenii Acuti,

Radix Achyrantis Bidentatae, Radix Codonopsis Pilosulae

Indications: Wind in the channels and connecting vessels causing numbness and tingling of the hands and feet, soreness and pain of the low back and knees, lack of strength of the sinews and bones, difficulty walking

Mu Gua Wan ★

Ingredients: Radix Achyrantis Bidentatae, Radix Angelicae Sinensis, Caulis Piperis, Fructus Chaenomelis Lagenariae, Radix Clemetidis Chinensis, Radix Ligustici Wallichii, Caulis Milletiae Jixueteng, Radix Angelicae, Radix Aconiti Chuanwu, Radix Aconiti Caowu, Rhizoma Cibotti Barometz, Radix Panacis Ginseng

Indications: Wind/cold/damp *bi*, soreness and pain of the entire body, numbness and tingling of the four extremities, lack of strength of the sinews and bones, difficulty walking

Comparison of the Above Formulas

Hu Gu Jiu dispels wind dampness and problems of the sinews and bones due to kidney emptiness and invasion by wind dampness. In particular it is effective for low back pain, soreness of the legs and knees, and numbness and tingling of the four extremities.

Tian Ma Wan dispels wind dampness at the same times as it boosts the kidneys and strengthens the low back, nourishes the blood, and soothes the sinews. It is indicated for wind damp low back and knee soreness and pain, numbness and tingling of the four extremities, difficulty walking, inability to bend and stretch, etc.

137

Guo Gong Jiu treats wind dampness, nourishes the blood, and frees the connecting vessels. It is indicated for numbness and tingling of the four extremities due to wind dampness, discomfort of arms and legs, and inhibition of the joints.

Hu Gu Mu Gua Wan and *Mu Gua Wan* both dispel wind dampness, strengthen the sinews and bones, disperse cold, and stop pain. They are indicated for the treatment of wind damp *bi* and pain accompanied by cold evils, soreness of the body with prominent dampness, numbness and tingling of the body and limbs, and difficulty walking.

2. Dispelling Wind Dampness, Freeing the Channels & Connecting Vessels, Dispersing Cold & Stopping Pain

The following patent medicines dispel wind and eliminate dampness, activate the blood and free the connecting vessels, disperse cold and stop pain. As a group they are indicated for the treatment of wind damp *bi* and pain, inhibition of the joints, numbness and tingling of the body and extremities, and other similar conditions. In addition, they supplement, boost, and support the righteous.

Wu Jia Pi Jiu ★

Ingredients: Radix Angelicae Sinensis, Rhizoma Sinomenii Acuti, Radix Ligustici Wallichii, Radix Clemetidis Chinensis, Fructus Chenomelis Lagenariae, Rhizoma Atractylodis Macrocephalae, Radix Angelicae, Radix Achyrantis Bidentatae, Flos Carthami, Cortex Radicis Acanthopanacis, Radix Codonopsis Pilosulae, Rhizoma Curcumae, Radix Angelicae Duhuo, Radix Aconiti Chaunwu, Radix Aconiti Caowu, Rhizoma Polygonati, Semen Myristicae Fragrantis, Lignum Santali Albi, Flos

Chrysanthemi, Flos Caryophylli, Fructus Seu Semen Amomi, Fructus Amomi Cardamomi, Radix Saussureae Seu Vladimiriae, Pericarpium Citri Reticulatae, Cortex Cinnamomi, Fructus Gardeniae Jasminoidis, white sugar, grain alcohol

Indications: Wind dampness causing spasms of the hands and feet, numbness and tingling of the four extremities, soreness and pain of the low back and knees, in men a damp scrotum and in women a chilly vagina (i.e., frigidity)

Feng Shi Guan Jie Jiu ★

Ingredients: Radix Achyranthis Bidentatae, Radix Ledebouriellae Sesloidis, Fructus Chaenomelis Lagenariae, Radix Et Rhizoma Notoptergyii, Radix Clemetidis Chinensis, Radix Aconiti Caowu, Ramulus Cinnamomi, Lignum Pini Nodi, Radix Ligustici Wallichii, Caulis Milletiae Jixueteng, Radix Angelicae Sinensis, Rhizoma Atractylodis, Rhizoma Dioscoreae Nipponicae, Zaocys Dhumnades, Radix Alba Paeoniae Lactiflorae, Fructus Citri Sacrodactylis, Radix Panacis Ginseng, Radix Glycyrrhizae, Herba Bidentis Bipinnatae, Cortex Radicis Acanthopanacis, Rhizoma Dioscoreae Bixie Seu Hypoglaucae, Radix Angelicae Duhuo, Semen Fermentatus Cum Monasconim Oryzae, brown sugar, grain alcohol

Indications: Wind dampness inflammation of the joints, soreness and pain of the joints, shoulder pain, numbness and tingling of the four extremities, low back pain and coldness of the knees, inflexibility of the sinews and vessels

Shu Feng Ding Tong Wan ★

Ingredients: Herba Ephedrae, Olibanum, Myrrha, Rhizoma Homalomenae Occultae, Radix Schizophragmae Integrifoliae,

Ramulus Cinnamomi, Radix Achyranthis Bidentatae, Fructus Chaenomelis Lagenariae, Pyritum, Radix Glycyrrhizae, fresh Cortex Eucommiae Ulmoidis, Radix Ledebouriellae Sesloidis, Radix Et Rhizoma Notopterygii, Radix Angelicae Duhuo, Pulvis Semenis Strychnotis

Indications: Attack by wind and cold, joint soreness and pain, sinews and connecting vessels not relaxed, numbness and tingling of the four extremities, weakness and pain of the low back and knees, lack of strength of the legs and knees; also good for injury and trauma

San She Dan Zhi Jiu ★

Ingredients: Cortex Eucommiae Ulmoidis, Radix Angelicae Sinensis, Radix Achyranthis Bidentatae, liquid juice from trio of snake gallbladders, Nidus Vespae

Indications: Wind dampness *bi* and pain, inhibition of sinews and bones, soreness and pain of the low back and knees, flaccid weakness of the lower extremities, etc.

Comparison of the Above Formulas

Wu Jia Pi Jiu eliminates dampness and dispels wind, soothes the sinews and activates the blood in the treatment of wind dampness with low back and knee soreness, damp scrotum in men and chilly vagina (*yin leng*) or frigidity in women.

Feng Shi Guan Jie Jiu rids cold, disperses wind, eliminates dampness, and activates the blood in the treatment of wind damp pain with more pronounced cold.

Shu Feng Ding Tong Wan dispels wind and disperses cold, activates the blood and stops pain, extinguishes wind and stops pain in the treatment of wind dampness with more obvious dampness and also in trauma and injury.

San She Dan Zhi Jiu dispels wind dampness and relaxes the sinews and connecting vessels at the same time that it nourishes, tonifies, and strengthens. It is indicated for the treatment of wind dampness with soreness and pain of the low back and knees, lack of strength and flaccid weakness of the lower extremities, and difficulty walking.

3. External Medications for Dispelling Wind & Dispersing Cold, Activating the Blood & Stopping Pain

The two externally applied medicinal plasters described below dispel wind, disperse cold, and stop pain.

Gou Pi Gao ★♦

Ingredients: Fructus Immaturus Citri Seu Ponciri, Pericarpium Viridis Citri Reticulatae, Semen Hydnocarpi Anthelminthicae, Hallyositum Rubrum, Radix Rubra Paeoniae Lactiflorae, Rhizoma Gastrodiae Elatae, Radix Glycyrrhizae, Radix Linderae Strychnifoliae, Radix Achyranthis Bidentatae, Radix Et Rhizoma Notopterygii, Cortex Phellodendri, Fructus Psoraleae Corylifoliae, Radix Clemetidis Chinensis, fresh Radix Aconiti Chuanwu, Radix Saussureae Seu Vladimiriae, Radix Dipsaci, Radix Morindae Officinalis, Semen Pruni Persicae, Radix Praeparatus Aconiti Carmichaeli, Radix Ligustici Wallichii, fresh Radix Aconiti Caowu, fresh Cortex Eucommiae Ulmoidis, Radix Polygalae Tenuifoliae, Squama Manitis, Rhizoma Cyperi Rotundi, Rhizoma Atractylodis Macrocephalae, Semen Zanthoxyli Bungeani, Lignum Santali Albi, Fructus Foeniculi Vulgaris, Semen Cnidii Monnieri, Radix Angelicae Sinensis, Herba Cum Radice Asari, Semen Cuscutae, Pericar-

141

pium Citri Reticulatae, Rhizoma Sinomeii Acuti, Acacia Catechu, Flos Caryophylli, Myrrha, Sanguis Draconis, Olibanum, Cortex Cinnamomi, Calomelas, Camphora

Indications: Wind/damp/warm *bi* causing low back soreness and pain, numbness and tingling of the extremities, and external injuries and trauma

Zhui Feng Gao ★

Ingredients: Radix Achyranthis Bidentatae, Semen Pruni Persicae, Herba Ephedrae, Radix Angelicae Sinensis, fresh Radix Aconiti Caowu, Herba Cirsii Japonici, Rhizoma Gastrodiae Elatae, Radix Angelicae Duhuo, Squama Manitis, Herba Cum Radice Asari, Radix Linderae Strychnifoliae, Radix Angelicae, Rhizoma Alpiniae Offinciari, Radix Et Rhizoma Notopterygii, Radix Rubra Paeoniae Lactiflorae, Rhizoma Sinomenii Acuti, Flos Carthami, Periostracum Serpentis, Lignum Sappan, Scolopendra Subspinipes, Radix Clemetidis Chinensis, Radix Rehmanniae, Radix Conquita Rehmanniae, Radix Aconiti Chuanwu, Radix Dipsaci, Cortex Radicis Acanthopanacis, Cortex Cinnamomi, Olibanum, Myrrha, Pollen Typhae, Lignum Santali Albi, Sanguis Draconis, Flos Caryophylli, Secretio Moschi Moschiferi, Borneolum

Indications: Wind damp soreness and pain of the sinews and bones, numbness and tingling of the four extremities, lumbar and backache, difficulty walking.

Comparison of the Above Formulas

Gou Pi Gao and *Zhui Feng Gao* are both externally applied, medicinal plasters. *Gou Pi Gao* is for the treatment of wind dampness causing pain of the joints and also is good for traumatic injuries. *Zhui Feng Gao* chases wind, disperses cold, soothes the sinews, and activates the blood in the treatment of wind cold causing numbness and tingling of the body and extremities, soreness and pain, inhibition of bending and stretching, and other similar conditions.

XV. Trauma & Injury Due to Strike & Fall

Because of decline of qi and blood and diminishment of strength, the elderly are prone to falling. Concomitantly, also because of decline of qi and blood, their circulation also tend to be retarded. Therefore, the elderly do not recuperate as quickly from traumatic injuries as fast as those younger. In addition, because of insufficiency of *jing* and blood the sinews tend to be stiff and inflexible and the bones weak and brittle and, therefore, more easily damaged in the aged.

If traumatic injuries go untreated and unhealed, acute injuries may give rise to chronic pain and disease. This is especially so in older persons. For this reason, it is especially important to treated quickly any traumatic injuries. The patent medicines described below are all for the treatment of trauma and injury due to fall and strike. As a group, they activate the blood, dispel stagnation, disperse swelling, and stop pain.

Yun Nan Bai Yao ★♦

Ingredients: Radix Pseudoginseng, Secretio Moschi Moschiferi, Radix Aconiti Caowu, etc.

Indications: Traumatic injuries and hemorrhagic disorders, gynecological hemorrhagic conditions, peptic ulcers and chronic stomach pain, and sore, swollen throat

143

Die Da Wan ★♦

Ingredients: Radix Angelicae Sinensis, Radix Ligustici Wallichii, Eupolyphagae Seu Opisthoplatiae, Sanguis Draconis, Myrrha, Herba Ephedrae, Olibanum, Secretio Moschi Moschiferi, Pyritum, Semen Strychnotis

Indications: Traumatic injury due to fall and strike, swelling and purpling of the skin, injuries of the sinews and bones, lumbar soreness and pain due to blood stagnation, and pain in the chest when breathing due to low back twist

Qi Li San ★♦

Ingredients: Sanguis Draconis, Flos Carthami, Acacia Catechu, Olibanum, Myrrha, Secretio Moschi Moschiferi, Borneolum, Cinnabaris

Indications: Traumatic injury, pain in the chest when breathing due to low back twist, bleeding due to incised wound, and pain due to stagnant blood

Yao Tong Wan ★

Ingredients: *Ji Xiang Cao* (identification unknown), *Shan Ju* (identification unknown), Fructus Psoraleae Corylifoliae, Radix Achyranthis Bidentatae, Radix Dioscoreae Oppositae, Radix Dipsaci

Indications: Twist, fall, or wrenching injury, and acute or chronic low back pain

144

XVI. Ulcers, Boils, Swellings, & Hemorrhoids

The majority of boils, ulcers, and swellings belong to the heat category. When boils and ulcers are red in color, swollen, hot, and painful, they are typically accompanied by other signs of heat, such as fever, thirst, dry stool, and red urine. In such cases, one needs to clear heat, dissolve toxins, cool the blood, and disperse swelling. If there is pus, one needs to clear heat, dry dampness, and eliminate pus.

However, in the weak and elderly, ulcers and swellings usually belong to the empty cold category as evidenced by normal skin color, absence of pus, and lack of redness and pain except when pressed, or ulcers which weep a clear, watery discharge. In this case, the treatment principles are to warm yang, free the vessels, boost the qi, and nourish the blood, eliminate phlegm, disperse nodulation, astringe the ulcer, and generate flesh.

Hemorrhoids are also a common problem amongst the elderly. Hemorrhoids are evidenced by a painful swelling around the anus, bleeding with defecation, and difficult defecation. These symptoms are due to fire and heat accumulating in the Large Intestine in which case it is necessary to cool the blood, Dissolve toxins, purge heat, and free the bowels. However, for the treatment of chronic hemorrhoids with prolapse of the anus and an empty, weak constitution, it is necessary to boost the qi and lift yang.

Lian Qiao Bai Du Wan ★♦

Ingredients: Fructus Forsythiae Suspensae, Flos Lonicerae Japonicae, Radix Et Rhizoma Rhei, Herba Cum Radice Taraxici Mongolici, Herba Cum Radice Violae, Radix Scutellariae Baicalensis, Fructus Gardeniae Jasminoidis, Radix

Angelicae, Bulbus Fritillariae, Radix Rubra Paeoniae Lactiflorae, Radix Platycodi Grandilfori, Caulis Akebiae Mutong, Radix Ledebouriellae Sesloidis, Cortex Radicis Dictamni, Radix Glycyrrhizae, Periostracum Cicadae, Radix Trichosanthis Kirlowii

Indications: Acute ulcers and boils with redness, swelling, heat, and pain, aversion to cold and fever, urination and defecation knotted and shut, wind damp swelling, lump, or boil, and itching of the entire body

Xiao Jin Dan ★

Ingredients: Resina Liquidambaris Taiwanianae, Lumbricus, Radix Angelicae Sinensis, Myrrha, Radix Aconiti Caowu, Feces Trogopterori Seu Pteromi, Olibanum, fragrant ink black (*Xiang Mo*), Semen Momordicae, Secretio Moschi Moschiferi

Indications: All types of toxic swellings, abscesses in the breasts, vaginal lesions, and toxic swellings of unknown etiology

Yang He Wan ★

Ingredients: Radix Conquita Rehmanniae, Semen Sinapis Albae, Herba Ephedrae, Cortex Cinnamomi, Rhizoma Desiccata Zingiberis, Radix Glycyrrhizae, Gelatinum Cornu Cervi

Indications: Empty cold ulcers and swellings, swellings without a head, normal skin color, absence of heat, watery discharge, pale tongue with white coating, no thirst, and a deep, thready or slow, thready pulse

Di Yu Huai Jiao Wan ★

Ingredients: Fructus Sophorae Japonicae, Flos Immaturus Sophorae Japonicae, Radix Carbonisatus Sanguisorbae Officinalis, Fructus Immaturus Citri Seu Ponciri, Flos Carthami, Radix Angelicae Sinensis, Radix Scutellariae Baicalensis, Radix Rehmanniae, Radix Et Rhizoma Rhei, Radix Rubra Paeoniae Lactiflorae, Radix Ledebouriellae Sesloidis, Herba Seu Flos Schizonepetae Tenuifoliae

Indications: Hemorrhoids due to full heat, flourishing of fire in the large intestine, intestinal wind with bloody stools, stagnant heat, and itching and pain of the anus

XVII. Zheng Jia Ji Ju, Masses, & Phlegm Stagnation

In the root text upon which this present work is based, there is a section on the treatment of various types of tumors. Tumors and especially malignant tumors are the bane of the elderly's existence. However, tumors, whether benign or malignant, are the province of another specialty within Traditional Chinese Medicine called *zhong liu ke. Zhong liu ke* roughly corresponds to oncology in Western medicine. It is generally a specialty reserved for the most experienced and highest levels of TCM practitioners. The TCM treatment of tumors usually makes use of very large formulas dispensed as freshly brewed decoctions. It is not uncommon to see prescriptions for cancer patients running to twenty or more individual ingredients and two to three hundred grams per day. In some cases, patent medicines are used as adjunctive therapy and as a way to simply get more medicine into the patient without making them drink even more and stronger decoctions.

147

饮食有节

忌暴饮暴食

Be abstinent in food and drink;
Refrain from eating and drinking till you bulge

Although none of the patent medicines described in this section of the main text are available in the United States and although the treatment of tumors typically requires much stronger medicine than such patent medicinals, we have chosen to translate the introductory paragraphs of this section in any case. They give some idea of how TCM categorizes tumors and the treatment principles generally employed in their treatment. In particular, this section also gives important advice for the prevention of such tumors in the elderly.

Zheng jia ji ju refers to various types of masses in the abdomen. *Zheng ji* refers to those which have a palpable form and which are not movable. If there is pain, that pain is fixed in location. Such masses are categorized as species of blood stagnation. *Jia ju*, on the other hand, are formless and migrating, and if there is pain, it is not fixed in location. These types of lumps or accumulations come and go and are a species of qi accumulation. For instance, enlargement of the liver and spleen accompanying such gynecological diseases as uterine myoma and ovarian cysts belongs to this category.

If there is longterm depression or improper diet, these may injury the liver and spleen and cause stagnation of the qi and blood. This gradually develops into various types of masses and is especially associated with emptiness of righteous qi. Therefore, to prevent *zheng jia ji ju* one needs to cultivate a better mood and avoid all emotional upset and depression. One should also strengthen their constitution and pay attention to achieving a healthy lifestyle. The therapeutic principles for treating abdominal masses categorized in Chinese medicine as *zheng jia ji ju* are to regulate the qi and disperse nodulation, activate the blood and disperse stagnation, and to soften hardness and disperse swellings.

Ying liu means goiter and tumors of the neck. It refers to enlargement of the thyroid and is also related to emotional upset. When one is extremely depressed, angry, or worried, the liver loses its spreading and dredging function which in turn results in liver qi stagnation and may further transform into fire. This fire may stew the juices and transform into phlegm which is then drafted up into the throat where it lodges. This phlegm qi stagnation may then transform into a mass. Therefore, one should try to keep a calm mood so as to avoid goiters and tumors of the neck and thyroid. Since dampness plays a part in this scenario (it is dampness which is brewed into phlegm), diet also plays a part in the creation of phlegm masses. The therapeutic principles for the treatment of goiters and thyroid tumors are to dredge the liver and regulate the qi, clear fire and transform phlegm, and soften hardness and disperse nodulation.

Tan he or phlegm pit or nodule refers to a swollen, hard lymph node under the chin, in the neck, front or back, in the axillae. This is due to stagnation of phlegm and dampness. The therapeutic principles for treating such phlegm nodules are to transform phlegm and disperse nodulation, clear heat and dissolve toxins.

In general, tumors or *zhong liu* are related to internal injury by the seven passions which disturb *zang fu* function and thus cause stagnation of phlegm, qi, and blood. Therefore, one should pay special attention to their emotions. The general principles for treating tumors are to crack the qi, transform stagnation, disperse phlegm, and scatter nodulation.

Patent Medicine Index
With Ideograms

152

156

General Index

abdominal bloating 7, 26, 39, 41-43
abdominal bloating after meals 39
abscesses 107, 146
acid regurgitation 128
amenorrhea 34
anemia 29, 30, 32, 34, 35, 50, 62
anger 11, 12, 17, 57, 79, 84, 121
anxiety 12
aphasia 84, 86
arms and legs, heaviness of the 134, 138
arteriosclerosis 19, 20, 74
arteritis 74, 76
asthma 7, 11, 20, 28, 31-33, 50, 89-95, 97, 98
atherosclerotic heart disease 72

backache 142
balding 29
bedsores 33
belching 12, 123, 125, 126
bi 66, 72, 85, 132-138, 140, 142
bitter taste 79-81, 101, 114
bleeding due to incised wound 20, 33, 55, 74, 84, 130, 131, 144, 145
bloating 7, 12, 19, 26, 39, 41-43
blood extreme 22
blood lin 130
bodily weariness 59
body aches and pains 99
boils 107, 145, 146
bone extreme 22
bone spurs 67
bone steaming heat 53, 54
bones and sinews without strength 55
bones weak and brittle 143
borborygmus 40
bowel movements which are not free flowing 124

bronchi, swollen 95
bronchial asthma 20, 89
bronchiectasis 89
bronchitis 31, 60, 62, 89, 93-97
bronchitis, chronic 97
brooding 11
burping 40

cancer 3, 12, 19, 30, 97, 147
carbuncles 107
cerebral angiospasm 15, 71, 84, 88
Chao Shi Bing Yuan 21
Chao's Source of Disease 21
chest fullness 121, 122
chest obstruction pain 72
chest pain 71, 72, 91
chi yan 110
childbirth 29
chilly jing 52
cholecystitis 20
cirrhosis 20
clear-eyed blindness 110
cold damp bi 66
cold extremities 38
coma 84, 85, 105, 106
common cold 95, 96, 98-100, 102, 103, 116
common cold with toxic condition 103
constipation 20, 37, 74, 81, 93, 104, 105, 107-109, 113, 114, 118-122, 128
coronary artery 19, 20, 60, 71, 74-77, 80, 83, 86
cough 7, 11, 28, 31, 33, 54, 61, 62, 89-101, 103
cough due to common cold 96
cough with profuse phlegm 94, 100
crying 11

cystitis 131

damp *bi* 66, 133, 134, 136-138
Dao 1, 2, 13, 16, 129
deafness 4, 8, 22, 23, 53, 68-70, 79
defecation knotted and shut 146
delirium 104-106
depression 12, 57, 91, 121, 123, 124, 149
desires 2, 17, 44, 118
diabetes 19, 20, 28, 37, 51, 53, 55, 56
diarrhea 20, 28, 40-44, 61, 83, 91, 101, 117, 118, 125, 126, 127, 128, 131
diet 2, 10, 12, 15, 18, 84, 117, 149, 150
dizziness 8, 12, 13, 23, 26-28, 31, 34, 35, 39, 47-50, 52, 53, 55, 60, 62-65, 68, 70, 76, 77, 79, 80, 81, 82, 85, 106, 110, 111, 113-115, 116
dry stool constipation 109

earache 81
edema 36, 101, 128-131
emaciation 22, 28, 91
emotional factors 11
emotional stress 12, 113
emotions 5, 11, 12, 17, 57, 84, 114, 150
emphysema 89, 98
encephalitis 84, 104, 105
epidemic diseases, acute 105
epistaxis 54, 62, 104
essence extreme 22
essence spirit taxation 51
exercise 2, 13, 15
external evils 16, 26, 45, 72, 76, 82, 84, 90, 99, 101-103, 112, 113, 115, 116, 131, 133, 141, 142

face and cheeks, red 79, 82, 113

fall and strike 14, 143, 144
fang lao 13
fat deposits 20
fat *lin* 130
fatigue 15, 20, 23, 26-28, 31, 33, 34, 39, 44, 45, 47-49, 51, 52, 58, 60, 61, 64, 65, 91, 100, 121, 126, 127
fear 11, 48, 52, 90, 99-102, 112, 116
fear of cold 52, 99-102, 116
fear of draft 100
fear of wind 90, 112
fever 42, 76, 85, 90, 92, 94, 96, 98-106, 113, 115, 116, 131, 134, 145, 146
fire eyes 110
five colors 6
five taxations 21
flaccidity conditions 68
flesh extreme 22
forgetfulness 28, 33, 34, 48-50, 53, 57-60, 64, 80, 132
Fratkin, Jake viii
fright 11, 22
frigidity 139, 140
fullness after eating 5, 23, 40, 43, 68, 69, 91, 101, 115, 121, 122-125, 127, 128
furuncles 107

gao lin 130
glaucoma 111
goiter 149
gu ji 22
gynecological disorders 34

headache 28, 31, 34, 41, 64, 69, 76, 77, 79-81, 85, 92, 99, 101, 103, 112-116, 131
hearing problems 68
heart disease 3, 19, 29, 30, 60, 71, 72, 74-77, 80, 83, 86, 118

heartburn 60
heat in the center of the hands and feet 53, 65, 92
heat in the rectum 117
heatstroke 105
Heavenly decreed span 2
hematemesis 93
hemiplegia 84-87
hemoptysis 54, 93, 96, 104
hemorrhagic disorders 76, 144
hemorrhoids 145, 147
hepatitis 29, 30, 104
hernia 128
high blood pressure 20, 83
huo yan 110
hypercholesteremia 77
hypermenorrhea 74
hypertension 17, 19, 32, 53, 76, 77, 80, 82, 83, 115, 116, 118
hyperthyroidism 53

illness, chronic 28
impotence 8, 13, 28, 31, 34, 35, 38, 45, 47-52
incontinence of urine 47, 73
inguinal region, pain and distention of the 128
insomnia 6, 12, 14, 20, 28, 31, 32, 34, 35, 46-49, 57-65, 69, 70, 79, 80, 91, 92, 107, 114, 120
intercostal neuralgia 72
internal injury 44, 45, 53, 55, 56, 74, 77, 79, 85, 97, 101, 103, 109, 111-114, 130, 131, 150
inversion heart pain 72
irritability 53, 57, 79, 80, 91, 104, 105, 134
itching of the entire body 146

jaws and fists tightly clenched 85
jin ji 22

jing ji 22
joy 11, 12, 17
jue xin tong 72

kidney disease 53
knees and legs flaccid and weak 65

laryngitis 98, 99, 103
laughing 11
lethargy 26, 41, 114
leukemia 83
leukorrhea 34, 114
Li Guo-qing vii
Li Ma-kang 17
lifestyle 2, 9, 10, 13, 149
lin 47, 51, 129-132
lin zheng 129
liu ji 21
liu qi 10
liu xie 10
low back and knees, weakness and soreness of 13, 23, 33, 34, 35, 38, 45, 47-56, 60, 64-70, 79, 85, 88, 89, 114, 130, 135-142, 144
lumbar soreness and pain 144

malnutrition 30
masses in the abdomen 149
Mayway Trading Corporation vii
meningitis 104, 105
menopathies 34
menorrhagia 34, 74
mouth, dry 65
mucous flecked with blood 96
muscular strain 66, 67

nausea 28, 93, 101, 115, 121
Nei Jing 1, 8, 9, 13, 15, 16, 19, 112
nephrolithiasis 131
neuralgia 29, 72

neurasthenia 30, 32, 35, 58-61, 64, 115
neurological impairment 88
neurosis 115
night blindness 110
night sweats 32, 34, 49, 53-55, 70, 96, 97
nocturnal emissions 54
nodulation 145, 149, 150
Nuherbs Company vii
numbness 27, 85, 133, 134, 136-140, 142, 143

obesity 19, 20, 74, 83
oncology 147
osteophytes 67, 68
ovarian cysts 149
overtaxation by the seven passions 22
overthinking 12, 61

pain which migrates from joint to joint 133
pallor 22, 23, 27, 28, 33, 39, 40, 43, 50, 59, 65, 73, 85, 91, 100, 114
palpitations 6, 23, 26-28, 32-34, 50, 56-63, 69, 72, 73, 91, 107, 114, 120
Paradigm Publications viii, ix
paralysis, facial 106
peptic ulcers 144
periods, irregular 34
phlegm asthma 94
phlegm pit 150
photophobia 110
pi mao 99
pneumonia 89, 94, 96
polyuria 8, 28, 35, 51, 119, 131, 132
post partum weakness 34
post urination dribbling 128
prestroke conditions 87
prolapse of middle qi 36, 39, 40, 42, 43, 145

prostate gland 51, 129
pus 145

qi extreme 22
Qi Gong 15
qi ji 22
qi shang 21, 22
qing mang 110

red eyes 76, 81, 109, 110, 112, 120
regurgitation 40, 128
respiratory diseases 3, 98
rest 2, 13-15
rheumatoid arthritis 29, 30
rhinitis 115
rou ji 22

sadness 11, 12
salivation 55, 85
sallowness 59
sandy lin 130
scrotum damp and chilly 51
scrotum, swollen 49, 128
seizures 105
septicemia 104
seven injuries 21, 22
sex 9, 10, 12, 13, 45, 46, 84
sexual dysfunction 31
shan qi 128
Shen Lian-sheng vii
shock 61
shoulder pain 139
sighing 121
sinew extreme 22
six evils 10
six extremes 21, 22
six qi 10, 11
skin ulcers 33
Society for Respecting the Elderly 18
sore throat 53, 76, 90, 93, 99, 103,

Suppliers

Chinese Patent Medicines

Mayway Trading Co.
622 Broadway
San Francisco, CA 94133
(415) 788-3646
(800) 621-3646

Nuherbs Co.
3820 Penniman Ave.
Oakland, CA 94619
(415) 534-4372
(800) 233-4307
Fax (415) 534-4384

Powdered Extracts

Brion Herb CO.
9250 Jeronimo Rd.
Irvine, CA 92718
1-800-333-4372

Qualiherbs
13340 E. Firestone Blvd., Suite N
Santa Fe Springs, CA 90670
1-800-533-5907

ABOUT THE AUTHORS

Anna Lin, Lic.Ac., was born in Cambodia to a family with a long history of involvement with Traditional Chinese Medicine. Her first experiences with the art of Chinese medicine came at a very early age as an apprentice to a Dr. Ma in Saigon, Vietnam. Later she studied at the Guangzhou College of Traditional Chinese Medicine in the People's Republic of China and interned at Guangzhou TCM Hospital and Xia Men TCM Hospital. She also has a degree in literature and languages from Jinan University in Guangzhou.

During the 1980's Anna Lin practiced acupuncture and Chinese medicine in New Mexico, during which time she also received her MA in American Studies. She currently has a private practice in Torrance, CA and is the chief acupuncturist at Bayshore Medical Group. She is also an instructor at SAMRA Univeristy of Oriental Medicine.

Bob Flaws, DOM, CMT, Dipl.Ac., is an internationally known practitioner of and author on traditional Chinese medicine. He has written, translated, and edited over a dozen books on various aspects of Oriental medicine and numerous articles by Dr. Flaws have appeared in professional journals both in America and abroad. In addition, Dr. Flaws regularly lectures at many of the major American colleges of acupuncture and Oriental medicine and has been an invited speaker at several national and international medical conferences. His other credits include founding Blue Poppy Press.

Dr. Flaws originally studied acupuncture with Dr. Tao Xi-yu and at the Shanghai College of Traditional Chinese Medicine where he also studied Chinese herbal medicine and Tuina Chinese remedial massage. He is a founding member and past member of the Board of Directors of the Acupuncture Association of Colorado, a member of the American Association of Acupuncture and Oriental Medicine, was appointed a Research Associate of the Tibetan Medical Society, and is a graduate of the Boulder School of Massage Therapy. Since 1980, Dr. Flaws has conducted a private practice in traditional Chinese medicine in Boulder, CO.

OTHER BOOKS ON CHINESE MEDICINE AVAILABLE FROM BLUE POPPY PRESS

1775 Linden Ave
Boulder, CO 80304
303\442-0796

PMS: Its Cause, Diagnosis & Treatment According to Traditional Chinese Medicine by Bob Flaws ISBN 0-936185-22-8 $14.95

SOMETHING OLD, SOMETHING NEW; Essays on the TCM Description of Western Herbs, Pharmaceuticals, Vitamins & MInerals by Bob Flaws ISBN 0-936185-21-X $19.95

SCATOLOGY & THE GATE OF LIFE: The Role of the Large Intestine in Immunity, An Integrated Chinese-Western Approach by Bob Flaws ISBN 0-936185-20-1 $12.95

SECOND SPRING: A Guide To Healthy Menopause Through Traditional Chinese Medicine by Honora Lee Wolfe ISBN 0-936185-18-X $14.95

MIGRAINES & TRADITIONAL CHINESE MEDICINE: A Layperson's Guide by Bob Flaws ISBN 0-936185-15-5 $11.95

STICKING TO THE POINT: A Rational Methodology for the Step by Step Formulation & Administration of an Acupuncture Treatment by Bob Flaws ISBN 0-936185-17-1 $14.95

ENDOMETRIOSIS & INFERTILITY AND TRADITIONAL CHINESE MEDICINE: A Laywoman's Guide by Bob Flaws ISBN 0-936185-14-7 $9.95

CLASSICAL MOXIBUSTION SKILLS IN CONTEMPORARY CLINICAL PRACTICE by Sung Baek ISBN 0-936185-16-3 $10.95

THE BREAST CONNECTION: A Laywoman's Guide to the Treatment of Breast Disease by Chinese Medicine by Honora Lee Wolfe ISBN 0-936185-13-9 $8.95

NINE OUNCES: A Nine Part Program For The Prevention of AIDS in HIV Positive Persons by Bob Flaws ISBN

0-936185-12-0 $9.95

THE TREATMENT OF CANCER BY INTEGRATED CHINESE-WESTERN MEDICINE by Zhang Dai-zhao, trans. by Zhang Ting-liang & Bob Flaws, ISBN 0-936185-11-2 $16.95

BLUE POPPY ESSAYS: 1988 Translations and Ruminations on Chinese Medicine by Flaws, Chace et al, ISBN 0-936185-10-4 $18.95

A HANDBOOK OF TRADITIONAL CHINESE DERMATOLOGY by Liang Jian-hui, trans. by Zhang Ting-liang & Bob Flaws, ISBN 0-936185-07-4 $14.95

SECRET SHAOLIN FORMULAE FOR THE TREATMENT OF EXTERNAL INJURY by Patriarch De Chan, trans. by Zhang Ting-liang & Bob Flaws, ISBN 0-936185-08-2 $13.95

A HANDBOOK OF TRADITIONAL CHINESE GYNECOLOGY by Zhejiang College of TCM, trans. by Zhang Ting-liang, ISBN 0-936185-06-6 $17.95

FREE & EASY: Traditional Chinese Gynecology for American Women 2nd Edition, by Bob Flaws, ISBN 0-936185-05-8 $15.95

PRINCE WEN HUI'S COOK: Chinese Dietary Therapy by Bob Flaws & Honora Lee Wolfe, ISBN 0-912111-05-4, $12.95 (Published by Paradigm Press, Brookline, MA)

TURTLE TAIL & OTHER TENDER MERCIES: Traditional Chinese Pediatrics by Bob Flaws ISBN 0-936185-00-7 $14.95

Against the Grain

Ian McMillan

Thomas Nelson and Sons Ltd
Nelson House   Mayfield Road
Walton-on-Thames   Surrey
KT12 5PL   UK

51 York Place
Edinburgh
EH1 3JD   UK

Thomas Nelson (Hong Kong) Ltd
Toppan Building 10/F
22A Westlands Road
Quarry Bay   Hong Kong

Thomas Nelson Australia
480 La Trobe Street
Melbourne   Victoria 3000
Australia

Nelson Canada
1120 Birchmount Road
Scarborough   Ontario
M1K 5G4   Canada

© Selection and editorial content copyright Ian McMillan 1989

Illustrations:

Cover photograph - Anthony Richardson
Section one - Pia Mobouck
Section two - Angela Duffy
Section three - Tilmann Walzer
Section four - Dandy Palmer
Section five - Louise Jackson
Section six - Sabine Tagwerker

First published by Thomas Nelson & Sons Ltd 1989

ISBN 0-17-432310-7
NPN 9 8 7 6 5 4 3 2 1

Printed in Great Britain by Scotprint Ltd,
Musselburgh, Scotland

Nelson

CONTENTS

INTRODUCTION

Hello. Welcome to *Against the Grain*. I hope you
enjoy some, or even all, of the poems in this book.
They don't pretend to be the best poems written in
the twentieth century, or the most important. They
are poems that I like. Poems that I wish had been
around in schoolbooks when I was beginning to
read and write poetry in secondary school many
years ago.

Enjoy is the key word in this book, closely
followed by *celebrate* and *rejoice*; these are not
poems to be taken apart and left for dead on a
wooden slab. Take them apart by all means . . .
borrow lines from them for your own poems;
borrow ideas, titles; write poems in reply to them.
Remember, *you* complete the poem by reading it.

I've divided the poems in the book into sections,
and at the end of each section I'll stand up and say
a few words. Maybe they'll be about why I like a
particular poem, or what a poem reminds me of.
Maybe I'll suggest some ideas for your own
writing or tell you anecdotes from my early life in
South Yorkshire.

Remember this, too: all poems are important,
from the poem written by a four year old to the
poem by the winner of the Nobel Prize for
Literature. Poems can be of all sorts: steps towards
self-discovery, battlecries, love letters . . . they can
even be poems.

Good reading, and good writing.

Ian McMillan

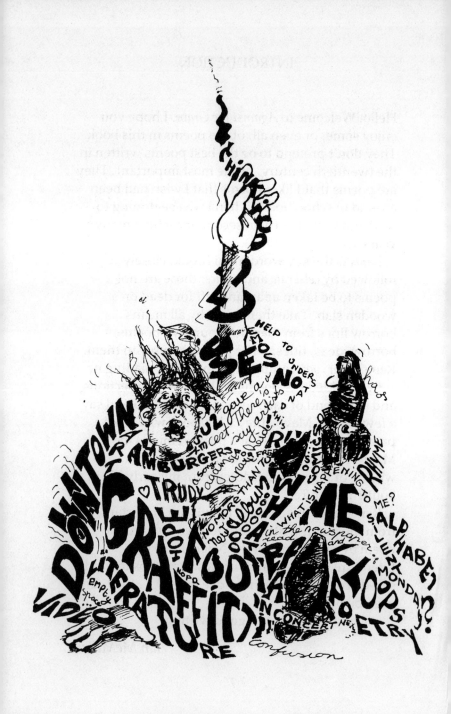

SECTION ONE

Brombistle Bay

To feast millicently
where nuthers acrease
in doolfastedly mingoes.
Suppance late folloy
inder wilberdreme
much haveringham gravels,
for doonseil mittens
searching lizendy upwards
wike oomblast sinnens.

Geoff Lowe

The Gift

My parcel was delivered to the college
Thoroughly packaged, like an only child . . .
I tear my father's beautifully written note
(*Please acknowledge receipt, Love Mum & Dad*)
Then fold the wrapping for possible re-use.
A breeze laps the posters crusting the wall;
Like lily pads, they compete to face the light.

I bump into Philip inside the Lodge.
He asks to see the gift – another four-sleeved
Pullover! Raising it shoulder-high, he
Teases me about the additional arms
Till I make my excuses and leave him
At the pigeonholes to scurry to my room.

I lay the jumper on my coverlet
And step back to survey the lively design –
Summery shades of green and blue in bars
A centimetre wide around the middle;
And seagulls, too. Trying it on before
My full-length mirror, I turn in circles like
A weather vane. The sleeves rotate with me!

Dizzier than Lewis Carroll's Alice, I
Finish instead an essay due at six . . .
My sides itch as I write. Just below the ribs,
Above my pelvis, carpal bones, knuckles,
And ten fingernails push through the flesh like roots.
Should I telephone home, or should I wait?

Stephen Knight

11

Concerning "The Flat of the Land"

I had this poem
that started out being about
the blue sky.

Then a lot of people popped up in this poem.

So I had this poem about a lot of people
under a blue sky.

Then all my friends wanted to be in it.

I said, "But there are a lot of people
in this poem already!"

"But we're your friends," they said.

So I had this poem about a lot of people
including all my friends
under a blue sky.

Then I put some weather in it
because it was a British poem.

Then I put place in it
because I remembered that
people need place.

So I had this poem about a lot of people
including all my friends
under a blue sky
in some weather
at a particular place.

The poem was no longer about the blue sky,
and I called it "The Flat of the Land".

"But nothing happens in this poem,"
I heard someone say. "It's so dull."

So,
I had this dull poem.

Martin Stannard

The Ingredient

Teacups have it.
I don't know why teacups have it,
but teacups do.
Horses turned out into a cold field have it,
as do the smouldering remains of a bonfire.
Mugs do not have it. That's a certainty.
Sacks of coal at the back gate have it,
and jig-saw puzzles have it,
and a river meandering through life has it.
A canal seems to have it, but it hasn't.
A bike has it, if it is a very very old bike.
Coloured pencils have it.
Leg irons are said to have it, but that's a joke,
and a very cruel joke at that.
This hasn't got it, but neither has a bottle of turps.
A Del Shannon 45 on the London label has it,
although a compilation LP of his Greatest Hits
doesn't have it even though it's tried really hard.
Ham salad has it.
Or rather, a ham salad can have it but it doesn't
    always.
Leather gauntlets have it, if they are brown leather
    gauntlets.
Discarded silk at the foot of the bed doesn't have it,
although sometimes it is worth pretending that it does.
Night has it, if it has been snowing.
The sea has it, even though it is saddened by oil,
and I am happy to live by the sea.
Aircraft do not have it.
Parks used to have it, but most have lost it

14

and are unlikely to regain that which has been
    squandered.
But ducks and swans have it. Especially swans.
And certain dreams have it.
Not all dreams, but certain dreams.
Some photographs have it.
Some photographs do not.
You do not have it, but not having it is not
    everything.
I rarely have it, and even when I do
it seems as if I am not quite myself.
Perhaps this explains how come teacups have it
and mugs do not.

Martin Stannard

Shadow on her Desk

A year after the courtroom heard those tapes
I'm running through the dark blue evening,
October fires keen on the wind, winter
    quickening.

In the tightening of fingers and the tightening of rules
something terrible was being hidden from us,
only the fear passed on, in rumour, safe at school.

Never take sweets from strangers (I'm running).
Don't accept lifts from people you don't know.
Better to be safe than sorry (I'm running).

That Friday I burst into a house doused with fish
my mother busy cooking, my father shushing me,
full of all my news my father shuts me up.

But I am shut before he says it,
seeing him crying, staring at the telly, crying.
Coal that burns in our grate has shut them up.

A slag heap, a tip, a shadow on her desk,
safe at school it shut them in the ground.
Safe at school it shut them.

After twenty years the one they tugged clear
stares out beyond the whirr of cameras to
the valley. Children gone, work gone,

only the green and the rain keep returning.
Fir trees are planted on man-made hills,
they've put up a memorial in pale cement.

After twenty years we are raking over old coals
but something terrible is being hidden from us,
only the fear passed on, in rumour, safe at school.

Don't play outside today (I'm crying).
Wash all green-leaved vegetables thoroughly.
Don't drink rainwater (I'm crying).

Saddleworth, Aberfan, Chernobyl: a kind of litany.
Up on the wet green moor police start to dig.

Maura Dooley

Elizabeth

(In the summer of 1968 thousands of people turned out
at the small stations along the route to see the train
carrying the body of Robert Kennedy from New York to
Arlington Memorial Cemetery in Washington. In
Elizabeth, New Jersey, three people were pressed
forward on to the line by the crowd and killed by a train
coming the other way – I happened to be travelling up
by the next train in this direction and passed the
bodies. One was of a black woman.)

Up from Philadelphia,
Kennedy on my mind,
Found you waiting in Elizabeth,
Lying there by the line.

Up from Philadelphia,
Wasn't going back,
Saw you, then saw your handbag
Forty yards on up the track.

Saw you under a blanket,
Black legs sticking through,
Thought a lot about Kennedy,
Thought a lot about you

Years later,

Blood on the line, blood on the line,
Elizabeth,
No end, no end to anything,
Nor any end to death.

No public grief by television,
Weeping all over town,
Nobody locked the train up
That struck the mourners down.

Nobody came to see you,
You weren't lying in state.
They swept you into a siding
And said the trains would be late.

They left you there in the siding
Against an outhouse wall
And the democratic primaries,
Oh they weren't affected at all,

In no way,

Blood on the line, blood on the line,
Elizabeth,
No end, no end to anything,
Nor any end to death.

Sirhan shot down Kennedy,
A bullet in L.A.,
But the one that broke Elizabeth,
It was coming the other way,

Coming on out of nowhere,
Into nowhere sped,
Blind as time, my darling,
Blind nothing in its head.

Elizabeth, Oh Elizabeth,
I cry your name and place
But you can't see under a blanket,
You can't see anyone's face,

Crying

Blood on the line, blood on the line,
Elizabeth,
No end, no end to anything,
Nor any end to death.

Kit Wright

And You Know What Thought Did

If you could eat frost, you might think
it would crunch like an apple. You might think

that it forms in fruit like a snowflake forms
in the air. Crisp, and clear. Not so.

Frost in the flesh of an apple runs soft
and brown, and in California they smoke it out

with stove-like affairs that burn wood,
oil, paraffin or coal. Strange then, that

Californian apples are so sweet; so fresh;
because if you could eat smoke you might think

it would taste like a kipper. Not frost.

Simon Armitage

Lizzie, Six

What are you doing?
I'm watching the moon.
I'll give you the moon
when I get up there.

Where are you going?
To play in the fields.
I'll give you fields,
bend over that chair.

What are you thinking?
I'm thinking of love.
I'll give you love
when I've climbed this stair.

Where are you hiding?
Deep in the wood.
I'll give you wood
when your bottom's bare.

Why are you crying?
I'm afraid of the dark.
I'll give you the dark
and I do not care.

Carol Ann Duffy

An Essay Justifying the Place of Science in the School Curriculum

Our physics teacher's Skullhead,
he's dead thin,
but has some dead good textbooks
with cartoons
where little men drop things
off blocks of flats.

Gravity is what
we did last week.

This morning Mrs Simpson
told me off
for having laddered tights
and said I must
appreciate the gravity
of crime.

Next week we're doing friction.
My mum thinks
that there is too much friction
in this world.

Chemistry we have
with Basher Bates.
We sit around his desk
while he does things
to litmus paper, it
goes red and green,
or is that colour blindness.

Well, this year
we have to choose our options
and I'd like
to do physics because
of the cartoons,
but can't because of chemistry
with Bates –
I'd have to take that too
you see, and Bates
once sent me out of class
because I laughed,
and laughing's not allowed
in chemistry.

Jane Hollinson

Like Strangers

Sometimes
Now he's come up from the Infants
I'll catch sight of my brother
At playtime in the playground
Playing Superman or Star Wars
With his best friend Stephen.

Sometimes
I'll be just chatting to Karen
They'll dash past without even
Noticing. Right beneath our
Noses yet they seem a million
Miles away. They could be

Strangers.
Like when I'll look down suddenly
And there's both my knees – as if
I'd never seen them before –
Between my sock tops and school skirt
After each holiday.

David Horner

Christmas Confessions

I'm telling you
they gave me a pasting.

Slammed mince pies
right into my belly.

Choked me on chocolates
plum puddings and brandy.

Aimed a great ham
right at my head.

It hit where it hurts
smack in the mouth.

They poked pork in my guts
made me an offer I couldn't refuse

concerning figs and satsumas
stilton and dates.

They poured beer and whisky
and wine down my throat.

"Hey!" they snarled
"spill the beans."

I'm telling you
I talked turkey.

David Harmer

Backwater

Fished him out, they did.

Who?

The bystanders.

No. Who was fished out?

The old boy.

What old boy?

The one who fell in.
The ice cracked.
Crowds gathered.
Touch and go it was.
Almost a panic.
Women screamed;
men shouted advice.

It was deep then?

No. Only up to his knees.
But it's a long time
since we've had
such excitement.

John Desmond

How Do/Who Me

got on a bus and saw
someone I once knew

and said How Do
and How Do said Who Me
and looked a bit funny at me
then got right off
whilst the bus was still stopped

Who Me I thought
How Do is still
as good a friend
as he was then

Geoff Lowe

Commentary

This section starts with 'Brombistle Bay' by Geoff
Lowe. I've chosen it as the first poem because it's
not the sort of poem you'd normally see as the first
poem in a book. I also chose it because I'm
intrigued by the noise it makes. Lots of nonsense
poems are pleasant and jolly. This one isn't; it's
got an unwieldy spiky sound that's just a bit
menacing. Try making up your own sound poems
with street names from your area, or racehorse
names from the newspaper, or your own name and
the names of the people in your class cut up and
thrown into the bin. 'Brombistle Bay' works very
well if you shout it out in a bus queue, by the way.

'The Gift' is a contrast: it looks like a poem, feels
like a poem. But what a strange story . . . maybe it
would work better as a story than a poem. Perhaps
it would make a good play, or a monologue, or
something. It's often worth looking at poems and
seeing if they'd work in other forms. Some poems
just work as poems. I can't imagine 'Brombistle
Bay' working as a nine-part television series for
Channel 4.

When I first read 'Concerning "The Flat of the
Land"', I turned the page to see if there was any
more, and of course there isn't. The ending
suggests more, and that has to be good in a world
where so many poems are far too long. I'm not
really sure what the poem's about, but I like the
way it appears to be about itself. I like the way
Martin Stannard has built the poem up. An old
Scottish word for poet is *Makar* . . . someone who

makes things. You can make poems like you can make cakes or brick walls . . . poems aren't found floating in mid air (not often, anyway!).

Here's another Martin Stannard poem. I suppose the question to ask about it is, "What is IT?" But I think another important question to ask is, "Does it matter if we don't know what IT is?" In other words, would the poem be spoiled for us if we knew what IT was? It would certainly be spoiled for me, but that doesn't mean it should be spoiled for you. It's only a list, really. So what makes it a poem?

Maura Dooley's 'Shadow on her Desk' explores the way we react to public events. A good workshop exercise is to write about a news item, and then write yourself into it, either as a detached observer, or as someone who is involved in the event. I realise that the events in the poem are history, but they're very much part of my personal history as well.

I don't want you to think that all the poems I like are strange and odd ones. 'Elizabeth' by Kit Wright tells a simple story in simple language, with good use of repetitions, which I like because repeating words and phrases is something you can do better in poetry than in prose.

I like poems with intriguing titles. The title of the poem has to act as a hook to drag the reader into the rest of the lines. 'Elizabeth' isn't a very exciting title, for instance. Sometimes titles can tell you too much. If you write a poem about memories, try not to call it 'Memories', because then we already know what the poem's about. Call it 'Fish on the Head' if it's about the time your grandad got a fish on his head as he was walking past the fish shop, and you'll make the reader want to read on. Call it 'The Day my Grandad got a Fish on his Head', and you'll be telling the reader that bit too much, I think.

'And You Know What Thought Did' is an intriguing title. When I was little we had a saying, "You know what thought did: he followed a muck cart and thought it was a wedding". Like many sayings from my childhood, it's more or less meaningless, but I *think* it means that if you're right, you're not, or something like that. I like the way that Simon Armitage ends lines on unimportant words like 'that' (which chimes in nicely on the page and in the head with words like 'soft', 'out' and 'frost'). Too often poems have lines where the whole rhythm and meaning rushes towards the last word; it makes the poem lean to one side. Of course, line endings like Simon Armitage's might feel arbitrary, might feel just like chopped-up prose. Do *you* think it feels like chopped-up prose? I don't, I think that each word has been balanced carefully and tested out before being used. But, if you do think it's chopped-up prose, is there anything wrong with that? It's worth getting a page of prose and trying to make a poem out of it by chopping up the lines.

'Lizzie, Six' is a frightening poem. It's to do, somehow, with the difference between expectation and reality. I expected, from the title (titles again: aren't they *important*?) to read a gentle poem about a little girl. Look at how simple the language is, and how tightly the poem is structured. For example: the middle lines end on the same word, the repeated 'ing' rhymes, and the successive 'air' sounds.

Of course, this book is about you writing your own poems as well as reading them. I hope the poems will give you ideas, give you starts for your own poems. A good way to start is by writing as though you're someone else. There's more about that in the 'Things to do' section at the end of the book.

'An Essay Justifying the Place of Science in the School Curriculum' isn't by a young schoolkid, but I think Jane Hollinson has captured a certain kind of pupil's voice very well. Do you think it's meant to be a boy or a girl? David Horner isn't, and never has been, a young girl, but in this poem 'Like Strangers', he writes as though he is a young girl. Do you think it works? If I hadn't told you, would you have expected it to have been written by a woman or a girl?

I hope that some of the poems in this section will make you want to go away and write poems as though you are Lord Nelson, or perhaps a young girl on the Isle of Mull in October 1923. October 5th, if you like. David Harmer isn't David Horner and he isn't a tough private detective from California, but in this poem 'Christmas Confessions' he's writing as though he is.

A variation on the poem in one voice, of course, is the poem in two voices. (Clever stuff, this; stick with me and you'll be on Mastermind!) 'Backwater' is an effective two-voice poem, set not too far away from the area Martin Stannard was describing in 'Concerning "The Flat of the Land"'. The last stanza of the poem has four lines. If I

altered it to a three line stanza, making "we've had
such excitement" the final line: do you think it
would work better?

The last poem in this section is here because
we've not been introduced properly yet. How do.

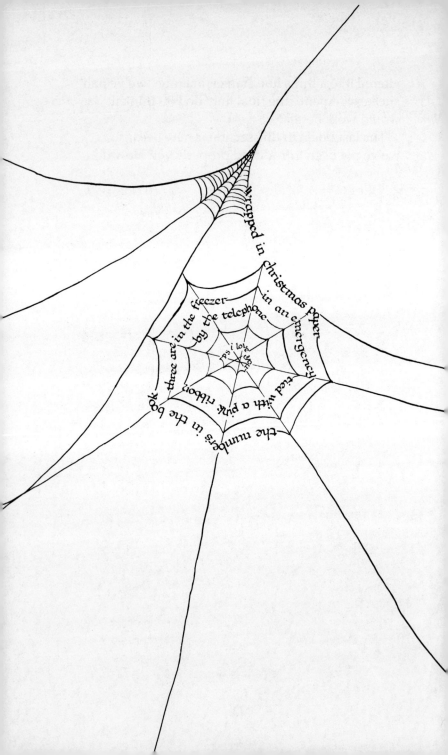

SECTION TWO

35

An Everyday Story of Countryfolk

Whenever anyone was killing a
pig, she would buy (they called her Pig Susie)
chitterlings, brains, blood, for a shilling a
bucketful. Married to the big, boozy
owner of the Glebe Farm, she nursed, in nine
years, eight children. Her black puddings and brawn
sustained them – bowls of brains immersed in brine
littered the kitchen like bowls of frog spawn.
    One evening, as she came from a neighbour's
with an apronful of pig guts, her man,
drunk from the Plough after his day's labours,
knocked her down with his bike. When she began
scraping the apron's contents up, poor bloke,
thinking he'd disembowelled her, had a stroke.

Peter Reading

Children

The children are playing a game of chase
and one of the children who seems to want to be
     chased after
calls out above the screams and laughter
don't chase me,
don't chase me!
and nobody does.

John Hegley

Children With Adults

My auntie gives me a colouring book and crayons.
I begin to colour.
After a while she looks over to see what I have
    done and says
you've gone over the lines
that's what you've done.
What do you think they're there for, ay?
Some kind of statement is it?
Going to be a rebel are we?
I begin to cry.
My uncle gives me a hanky and some blank paper
do your own designs he says
I begin to colour.
When I have done he looks over and tells me they
    are all very good.
He is lying,
only some of them are.

John Hegley

Mek Ah Ketch Har

Onoo hole mi yaw, onoo hole mi good,
No mek mi get weh do,
For ah mus kill har if mi ketch har,
Dat mawga gal name Sue.

Onoo no tell mi fe shet mo mout,
Ah mus sleep a jail tenite!
Long time now she dah fool roun mi,
An teday ah gwine bus a fight.

Look how de gal come lable mi,
Look how she call mi tief!
Jus' because she see mi a har kitchen
a tas'e har mah corn-beef.

An all a wi kno' har mah cyan cook,
so mi was jus' a try
see if mi coulda help dem out,
Mek sure de fat no dye.

For wi all memba las' Thursday nite
De hole o' dem nea'ly dead,
When dem done eat de tun corn-meal
Dem poison wid liquid lead.

Mi was jus' a try i' out,
Mek sure it was a'right,
Onoo let mi go mek a ketch har!
Dem gwine bury har before daylight.

Lawd! see har mah a come yah now!
Har pah a come wid har to!
Har brother, har sista an she herself,
A wha mi a go do?

Mercy! dem ha' one sobble-jack,
An one debbil ebba big crow-bar!
Mi done fah now, mi dead tenight,
A whey mi a go do Miss Flar?

Hide mi Miss Flar, hide mi,
No mek dem ketch mi please,
If dem ketch mi dem gwine kill mi
An yuh wi never be at ease.

A gawn dem gawn? Mi no see dem.
Dem 'fraid o' mi yuh kno'
Onoo let mi go mek a calla Sue!
Mek ah gi' har two big blow.

Ah gwine mek she kno' mi a big ooman,
A no yesterday mi bawn,
Lawd ha' massey, dem a come back,
Onoo gi mi pass, mi gawn!

Val Bloom

40

Dogs and Wolves

Across eternity, across its snows
I see my unwritten poems,
I see the spoor of their paws dappling
the untroubled whiteness of the snow:
bristles raging, bloody-tongued,
lean greyhounds and wolves
leaping over the tops of the dykes,
running under the shade of the trees of the wilderness
taking the defile of narrow glens,
making for the steepness of windy mountains;
their baying yell shrieking
across the hard barenesses of the terrible times,
their everlasting barking in my ears,
their onrush seizing my mind:
career of wolves and eerie dogs
swift in pursuit of the quarry,
through the forests without veering,
over the mountain tops without sheering;
the mild mad dogs of poetry,
wolves in chase of beauty,
beauty of soul and face,
a white deer over hills and plains,
the deer of your gentle beloved beauty,
a hunt without halt, without respite.

Sorley Maclean

41

Lion

My freend da lion his a waarm den.
Wi roar an grin, he bids da wind
Come in an fan his fire.
It døsna blaa oot,
But lowes still brichter,
Lichtin da mirk,
Still farder, still hicher.

We can aa øs dis lichthoose
I da broo, if we but open up
An coont da sowls itida mirk.
Dis nummers irna random,
Mind oot, dønna forgit dem,
Fir dey will be wir meid
Itida future.

We ir strang, no waek,
Pør, no wealty,
Soople, no stiff.

Let aa tochts be lichthooses,
Aa wyrds dir baems.
Hit isna as it seems,
Dis nummers irna random,
Dey ir wir meid.

Robert Alan Jamieson

Proverb (Tree Poem 4)

```
treetreetreetreetreetreetreetreetreetreetreetreetree
treetreetreetreetreetreetreetreetreetreetreetreetree
treetreetreetreetreetreetreetreetreetreetreetreetree
treetreetreetreetreetreetreetreetreetreetreetreetree
treetreetreetreetreetreetreetreetreetreetreetreetree
treetreetreetreetreetreetreetreetreetreetreetreetree
treetreetreetreetreetreetreetreetreetreetreetreetree
treetreetreetreetreetreetreetreetreetreetreetreetree
treetreetreetreetreetreetreetreetreetreetreetreetree
treetreetreetreetreetreetreetreetreetreetreetreetree
treetreetreetreetreetreetreetreetreetreetreetreetree
treetreetreetreetreetreetreetreetreetreetreetreetree
treetreetreetreetreetreewoodtreetreetreetreetreetree
treetreetreetreetreetreetreetreetreetreetreetreetree
treetreetreetreetreetreetreetreetreetreetreetreetree
treetreetreetreetreetreetreetreetreetreetreetreetree
treetreetreetreetreetreetreetreetreetreetreetreetree
treetreetreetreetreetreetreetreetreetreetreetreetree
treetreetreetreetreetreetreetreetreetreetreetreetree
treetreetreetreetreetreetreetreetreetreetreetreetree
treetreetreetreetreetreetreetreetreetreetreetreetree
treetreetreetreetreetreetreetreetreetreetreetreetree
treetreetreetreetreetreetreetreetreetreetreetreetree
treetreetreetreetreetreetreetreetreetreetreetreetree
treetreetreetreetreetreetreetreetreetreetreetreetree
```

Michael Gibbs

The Honey Pot

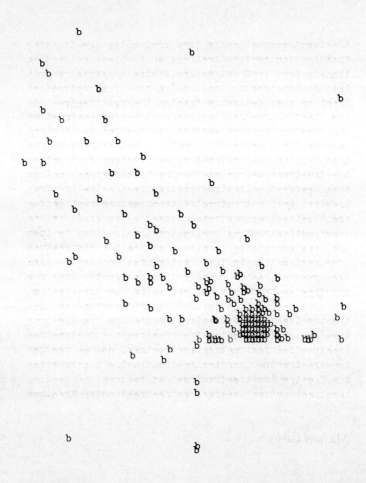

Alan Riddell

Zeeeyooosshhhhhhhh

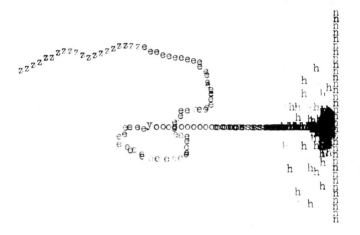

Cavan McCarthy

Danse Macabre

the tailor's fat wife
Silberhans, a minstrel
a stranger

a little girl, nine or ten years old
a younger girl, her little sister
a stranger

Weydenbusch, a senator
a student who knew many languages
a blind girl
the bailiff of Mergelsheim
a knife grinder
the woman who kept the bridge gate

a stranger

Alasdair Paterson

(*from a list of persons executed for witchcraft in the
                              bishopric of Würzburg*)

46

Using Obscene Language

His son killed mine he said
Using obscene language

Now I'm going to kill him he said
Using obscene language

He drove round to his house
Using obscene language

And broke down the door
Using obscene language

Where's your son he said
Using obscene language

I'm going to kill him he said
Using obscene language

They kept them apart
Using obscene language

I only meant to frighten him he said
Using obscene language

You've killed him he said
Using obscene language

An eye for an eye he said
Using obscene language

They took him away
Using obscene language

Now he's inside
Using obscene language

That's what happens
Using obscene language

Christine Herzberg

Singing in the Rain

Patient more stable than on my previous visit
although his mother reports he is often
abusive towards her.

Patient continues to spend his time
outside the home either walking or cycling;
he is often sullen and uncommunicative.

Patient's behaviour increasingly disturbed
frequently drinks to excess and spends hours
wandering the countryside; has taken up fishing.

Patients now staying in bed until lunchtime
says that people are getting at him
refuses to discuss his situation with me.

Patient claims to have seen a flying saucer
says that he knows how it works and that it
is piloted by men from the planet Blackpool.

Patient unwell today; was recently knocked
from his bicycle by a policecar, reported to have
become abusive and aggressive.

Patient has begun to wander the house at night
constantly goes up and down stairs disturbing his
mother and claiming omnipotence.

Patient has begun nocturnal singing
accompanying himself on a toy banjo,
yesterday he told his mother that she was

THE ALMIGHTY BASTARD and struck her
on the chest.
This morning patient admitted to hospital
under compulsory order.

Martyn Wiley

Admission

Three of us in an upstairs room,
the walls made of misty glass and
beyond is the ward where people move
with the silent deliberation of fish.

I look at my companion,
the doctor kissing his pipe
and my lady from the motorway bridge
her pockets full of shiny coal.

He tells her not to be afraid and
then begins the white coated questions
that tickle behind her eyes like magic feathers.

'What day is it today?'
'What month is it my dear?'
She twists a piece of string
'Do you know what year it is?'
Silence thickening.

The doctor lights his pipe and then
tries once more to touch her mind,
'My dear lady, do you see the clock on the wall,
please, could you tell me what time it is?'
Her head slowly turns, a windmill on a distant hill,
she smiles and whispers to me,
'Him a doctor and he can't even tell the time.'
Then she flies back to the safety of her head
and begins to empty her pockets of coal.

Martyn Wiley

Mrs Skinner, North Street

Milk bottles. Light through net. No post. Cat,
come here by the window, settle down. Morning
in the street awakes unwashed; a stale wind
breathing litter, last night's godlessness. This place
is hellbound in a handcart. Cat, you mark
my words. Strumpet. Slut. A different man
for every child and not a shred of shame.

My dentures grin at me, gargling water
on the mantelpiece. The days are gone
for smiling, wearing them to chatter down the road.
Good morning. Morning. Lovely day. Over the years
I've suffered loss, bereavement, loneliness.
A terrace of strangers. An old ghost
mouthing curses behind a cloudy, nylon veil.

Scrounger. Workshy. Cat, where is the world
I married; was carried into up a scrubbed stone step?
The young louts roam the neighbourhood.
Breaking of glass. Chants. Sour abuse of aerosols.
That social worker called me *xenophobic*. When she left,
I looked that word up. Fear, morbid dislike, of strangers.
Outside, the rain pours down relentlessly.

People scurry for shelter. How many hours
have I sat here, Cat, filled with bitterness
and knowing they'll none of them come?
Not till the day the smell is noticed.
Not till the day you're starving, Cat, and begin
to lick at my corpse. I twitch at this curtain
as the Asian man next door runs through the rain.

Carol Ann Duffy

On Vacation a Woman
Mistakes Her Leg

On vacation a woman mistakes her leg
for her husband's leg.

Perhaps the clock has been left behind
and an absence of daylight

inhabits the room like a stray that will not
be wakened. The bats come out, aimless

and maybe crazed with the sounds of air.
She wants her husband to fasten the screen.

He rises, walks awhile under the pines
and the moon, the legendary moon, asking himself

if he is brave. At dawn the invisible lake
glitters again. He guides the boat by the

sun, in circles, while she watches a line of trees
unravel behind his ear. Across the bay

a fisherman thinks they are watching
one another's lips, as he would do

if he were driving a lady in circles.
He thinks they are pink, and damp

with lotion under their flowered shirts.
They do not mention the clouds of shy minnows.

And later they step from bathing suits,
their false bodies on the pine floor.

Their windows pull the lake
right into the room. In their tumblers

the ice can be heard across a mile of water
where a farmer coming home notices the glass

animals his wife has set on the sill.

Leslie Ullman

From the Other Side of the Street

Does he know he shouldn't grasp your elbow,
cracked since Arizona
when I hit the power-brakes, hard,
and you smashed into the dashboard
giggling with pain?

Or that when your dream invades you,
and you stand at the window
drawing empty circles in the air,
shadows from the willow
on your throat,
he should wrap a heavy blanket
round your goose-flesh shoulders,
guide you, without speaking, to the wicker chair?

Does he know the scent of sawdust makes you sad,
and the rasp of broken glass
along a sandstone wall
fires crimson darts across your eyes,

and you're scared of yellow envelopes,

like to watch the sun through wine,

or stand beneath a tree in summer rain,
palm extended,
patient for the large drops,
falling slow,
to wash your lifeline,
flood the ravine
between your finger and your thumb?

Does he know how well you laugh
– snorting tea, one Sunday afternoon,
two twisting streams onto your lap,
when our youngest son complained
that the dog had drunk his tadpoles?

Or how quietly you cry
– when you couldn't sponge my screaming any more,
and you bit through the pillow,
a feather rising,
settling on your head?

Why don't you tell him
that he shouldn't grasp your elbow?

And why do you skip
as you swirl around the corner, out of sight?

John Latham

To the Spider in the Crevice Behind the Toilet Door

i have left you four flies
three are in the freezer next to the joint of beef
the other is wrapped in christmas paper
tied with a pink ribbon
beside the ironing table in the hall
should you need to contact me
in an emergency
the number's in the book
by the telephone.

p.s. i love you

Janet Sutherland

A Woman's Work

Will you forgive me that I did not run
to welcome you as you came in the door?
Forgive I did not sew your buttons on
and left a mess strewn on the kitchen floor?
A woman's work is never done
and there is more.

The things I did I should have left undone
the things I lost that I could not restore;
Will you forgive I wasn't any fun?
Will you forgive I couldn't give you more?
A woman's work is never done,
and there is more.

I never finished what I had begun,
I could not keep the promises I swore,
so we fought battles neither of us won
and I said, "Sorry!" and you banged the door.
A woman's work is never done
and there is more.

But in the empty space now you are gone
I find the time I didn't have before.
I lock the house and walk out to the sun
where the sea beats upon a wider shore
and woman's work is never done,
not any more.

Dorothy Nimmo

My Father's Hands

Nails like seashells,
rounded, salt-water
clean, skin smelling
disinfectant-sharp.

No car maintenance,
no gardening for such
hygenic hands, their
skills with mini-drills

untransferrable to
Black & Decker jobs
about the house. Yet
the wrists were strong

as steel-twisted rope.
'You need a good grip,'
he would say, yanking
on some reluctant tooth.

Such gentleness in
the stubby fingers when
he cradled a wounded
cheek, swabbed blood.

At the funeral they
gave thanks for those
hands. I bit back
tears, salt as his skin.

Moira Andrew

Tomorrow is Another Day

She left the kitchen tidy.
The rhubarb was in the pan
all cut up and ready to go.
I lifted the lid. The blanket
of sugar was red as Burgundy.

They had dressed Gran
in her cotton gown, the pink
eiderdown drawn up to her
chin. Cold, she was, all
living colour drained away.

Cotton wool wisped from
her lips. I longed to tuck
it in, to leave her looking
tidy. Her motto was to be
ready for every eventuality.

Clean knickers, will be in
the top drawer, white nightgown
wrapped in tissue paper.
She'd even wakened Grandpa
to tell him she was going.

'Phone Dolly,' she'd said,
organising the family to the
end. 'She'll find everything
ready for tomorrow's lunch.
Cold roast, rhubarb in the pan.'

Moira Andrew

Smoke Screen

Please don't mind, Grandad, if I stay at home today
but I'd rather lie in bed and close my eyes,

remembering the way you twirled your shiny shoe
when you taught me out-swing corners, in the park,

and your eyes grew young and dreamy
when you told how Plantagenet, your horse,

stopped his cart outside the Cholmondeley Arms
until you bought a gill of bitter, in a pail.

You see, we did cremations in Joan of Arc
at school. I couldn't bear to see your eyes

when the undertaker slides you from the coffin,
ropes you to the stake and strikes a match.

How can they watch you bravely burning
– kneeling round you on their hassocks

singing 'Onward Christian Soldiers',
while the purple music squeezes on your ears?

I want you with me at the bottom of the garden
in the soft sun before the dark,

measuring my height against your buttons
– last month, I'd only three to go.

When I told you that your eyes looked tired
and asked if you would die, you were quiet

for a while, then squeezed my knee. 'Not before
you score left-footed for West Brom', you said.

I know the flames can't hurt – you're like Shadrach
and those other men you sang to me about.

But you won't feel easy in the holy smoke
until it's so thick that they can't see you.

Then you'll loosen your bone collar-stud again.
But those eyes, Grandad. Those quiet eyes.

Are you wearing your best waistcoat
with a bag of all-sorts in your secret pocket?

John Latham

Cafe, Rainy Tuesday Morning

The boy keeps his cup of
dregs on the formica tabletop

in front of him as if
it were a ticket for admission.

He nurses it close to
his hands when the old man

comes clearing tables.
It's a white, semi-translucent

cup, the kind you always get
in cafes. People

go and come. But others
stay, like him. He's

not the only one. Today
he's got the table by the street.

He taps a wrinkled
cigarette made from the tin's dust.

The urn steams. The plateglass
steams. Again

he clears a segment
of it with his sleeve,

a windscreen-wiper's shape.
He's heading nowhere

fast, his father keeps on
telling him. He only knows it's slow,

too slow. It's not yet even
noon, and there's no future

in his tealeaves.
He bought *The Sun* this morning,

but it's rolled up
on the table near his cup. Now

and then absently he'll pick
it up and furl

it tighter in his two hands,
almost like you'd wring

a chicken's neck. The newsprint's
soiled

his fingers, but that's all
it's good for now. He

doesn't get it for the jobs. One
thing he's learning, that

it's hard to make a daily paper
last all day.

Duncan Bush

64

Pneumoconiosis

This is the dust:

black diamond dust.

I had thirty years in it, boy,
a laughing red mouth
coming up to spit smuts black
into a handkerchief.

But it's had forty years
in me now:
so fine
you could inhale it
through a gag.
I'll die with it now.
It's in me,
like my blued scars.

But I try not to think about it.

I take things pretty easy, these days;
one step at a time.
Especially the stairs.
I try not to think about it.

I saw my own brother: rising,
dying in panic, gasping
worse than a hooked carp
drowning in air.
Every breath was his last
till the last.

I try not to think about it. But

know me by my slow step,
the occasional little cough, involuntary
and delicate as a consumptive's,

and my lung full of budgerigars.

Duncan Bush

Boiled Egg Deluxe

1. Heat water in pan until it begins to bubble.

2. Add a tiny sprinkling of salt which will be
                                       absorbed through the shell.

3. Place egg on spoon and gently lower it into the water.

4. I said gently.

5. Whoops.

6. The soft white summer clouds come pillowing out.
                                       (poetry)

7. Whenever I am trying to crack an egg, I can't do it!

Gary Boswell

Commentary

I think it's important to test poems out by reading them aloud. It gives a different kind of life to the poem, fleshing it out, giving it a human dimension that poems can sometimes lack on the page. Read the one by Peter Reading aloud. What's your reaction? Mine was hysterical public laughter when I first read it in a bookshop in Shropshire, although I remember some people I read it to being sickened by it. It raises the old questions like: "What should we put in a poem?"; "Are there subjects that shouldn't go into poems?"; "Are there some ways of writing that you can't call poems, no matter how you try?". These are the questions that this anthology will fearlessly tackle. Well, maybe.

Some poems work better when read aloud. They are performance poems, written for a particular audience. In John Hegley's case, he writes for the alternative cabaret audience, and particularly, I think, for a London-based cabaret audience. These poems 'Children' and 'Children With Adults' are tightly written and rely on their punchline and an assumption that the audience is listening.

Val Bloom comes from Jamaica, and a lot of her poems are meant to be performed. 'Mek Ah Ketch Har' is very much a performance piece, and I find it odd that it's in strict four-line stanzas that don't really reflect the rhythm of the spoken word. The language is difficult for some people to understand, but it's fun trying to follow the clues –

it's rather like being a poetry detective!

It was in a big cold room in Edinburgh in 1985 that I heard the great Gaelic poet Sorley McLean read his work. Some he read in English, some in Gaelic. He read 'Dogs and Wolves' twice, in both languages. It was an unforgettable reading. It's in Shetlandic, the language of the Shetland Isles. Have a go at writing or performing a poem in a dialect or language from your area. If you've been told that your area hasn't got a dialect, invent one.

'The Honey Pot', 'Proverb (Tree Poem 4)' and 'Zeeeyooosshhhhhhhh' are, I suppose the opposite of performance poems. They're visual poems. These three are just puns, I guess. Are they poems, though? Whether they are or not, have a go at making some yourself with a typewriter. The best thing about poems like these is that they don't have a meaning. Isn't it a relief to get away from meaning?

Another type of poetry is the found poem. Here the poet isn't making the words up (do you ever make words up? Helobongle?), just collecting words that happen to be written elsewhere. There's a great deal of organisation of the words, particularly in the Alasdair Paterson poem 'Danse Macabre'. The words can, if you want, follow lots of the rules of poetry, except that you don't make them up. This poem by Christine Herzberg 'Using Obscene Language' is half a found poem: it was inspired by an item in the local paper about a violent attack where a lot of swearing was used. Instead of printing the rude words, the newspaper kept using the phrase "using obscene language", which forms the basis of the poem.

Once you decide that it doesn't matter if you borrow other people's words, and that the poetry police aren't going to come knocking at your door, then there are all sorts of things you can do with other people's phrases. 'Singing in the Rain' by Martyn Wiley uses actual words from case histories of the fifties. Except that sometimes he's altered the actual words to make them funnier, which is also something you're allowed to do. The poem questions our ideas about what is sane and sensible, and what isn't. Of course another way of 'finding' a poem is to write down exactly what happened . . .

Talking about found poems, I once found a poem when I was on holiday in the U.S.A. in 1977. Well, I didn't exactly find it. I bought it. I was down to my last dollar in Kennedy Airport, and I thought it would be a romantic, poetic gesture to spend it on a magazine called *The New Yorker*. I bought the magazine, and because of where I was and who I was (a dreamy fat man who was writing a poem a day), Leslie Ullman's 'On Vacation a Woman Mistakes Her Leg', which was printed in that copy, has remained my favourite poem of all time. I don't care if you don't like it. I love it. It's a poem on so many layers, and it taught me so much about line endings (as I've said before, you don't have to end a line on a strong word). It also showed me how poems don't have to be about anything specific, although I feel that there is a lot going on in the poem. Are the husband and wife happy? Is that farmer happy? Where are the children, if any?

In one sense I think the Leslie Ullman poem is a

love poem. People often write poems when they're in love, and that's often a mistake. If you've written love poems you might know what I mean. Some love poems work, though 'From the Other Side of the Street' is a lovely one by John Latham, which just lists things he knows about someone. It's true to say that you don't get many love poems about spiders, though.

Of course, love often dies, and all that people are left with is routine and drudgery. It's a hard task to write a poem about routine and drudgery without making it a routine poem. I think Dorothy Nimmo succeeds in 'A Woman's Work' because of the jaunty rhythm and simplicity of the poem.

'My Father's Hands', 'Tomorrow is Another Day' and 'Smoke Screen', are three poems about loved ones who have died. Like love, death is often written about, and the poems don't often work. I think these work because they stick to specific images about the loved person, rather than writing about abstract things.

Writing a poem about someone is an odd thing. It introduces you to the person being written about, and by the end of the poem you feel that you know them quite well. Obviously, the person may not be real, or may be a mixture of many people. I feel that the people written about by Duncan Bush in 'Pneumoconiosis' *are* real, but that could just be because I've known people like them. Look at the poem's last line. I think comparing a wheezy chest to the noise a budgie makes is brilliant. That's one of the functions of poetry, to startle with its language. Let's leave predictable language to notes for the milkman and newspaper reports.

Maybe an anthology of poems shouldn't be predictable, either. Here's a recipe for 'Boiled Egg Deluxe'!

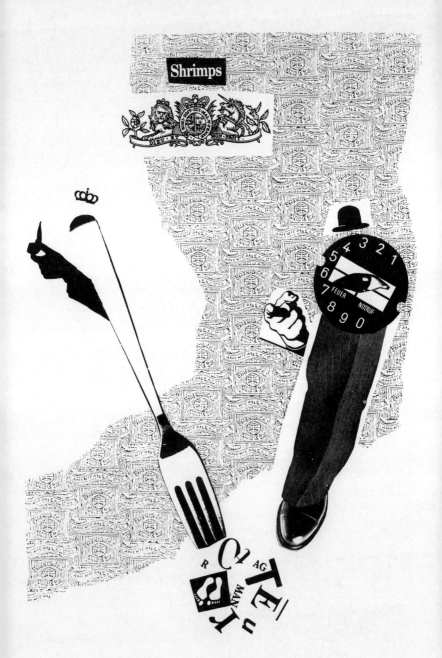

Shrimps

FEUER   NOTRUF

SECTION THREE

'Scouse Apache'

'Ang on a mo was a fearless warrior
'Ang on a mo was a ship-welder's mate,
'Ang on a mo worked at Cammell Laird's shipyard
'Ang on a mo never clocked on late –
You see, 'Ang on a mo had a squaw, two braves
    and a Japanese pinto.

'Ang on a mo bevied in the dingle
Teepeed in the florrie near the north end of town,
'Ang on a mo was a fearless warrior
'Ang on a mo never let his family down –
You see, 'Ang on a mo smoked the pipe of peace
    and made heap good music.

'Ang on a mo worked the great floating buffaloes
'Ang on a mo worked the great landing stage,
'Ang on a mo worked all the hours Manitoba sent him
'Ang on a mo sweated pelts to earn a wage, –
You see, 'Ang on a mo was put on a desert reservation
And all his warpaint and wahooing did him no good.

'Ang on a mo was a fearless warrior
'Ang on a mo was a spot welder's mate,
'Ang on a mo worked at Dunlop's factory;
'Ang on a mo
    hung himself on the Totem Pole near the gate.

Terry Caffrey

McCoy's Last Stand

Everyone on the back row
is reading, except Brown,
who is fishing for my attention:
he has his book upside down.

He is convincing. He leans forward
and turns a page, backwards.
I see the hook, but today
I am not biting. I am writing.

I imagine the denouement
in reverse: the hero's bullet
returns to his smoking gun
as the villain's blood spills uphill

and all the deeds are undone
as they eat their words:
"McCoy, surrounded is building whole the
up hands your with out come,"

but McCoy doesn't answer.
He's busy at the bank
handing money to the cashier.
The bell is ringing.

Duncan Curry

The Dirty Man

Roped up in his mac in a blackpaper parcel,
He stands till all hours in an entry without a gate
The parking light of his cigarette stub pulsing,
Frightening small girls but kicked by small boys
Returning from the Cubs or choir practice.
He slecks the dust on his path in a dry summer
With a pail of water and gives himself a lick and a
     promise,
Living off two lodgers dirtier than himself
And running credit up at the corner shop.
The other rainy evening I followed him
In the road at his own slow pace,
Getting to feel as vegetable as he must
To the point of not putting my umbrella up
And almost joining the bus queue as he does
For the sake of hearing some conversation.

Stanley Cook

A Novel

Doris is about to enter a convent.
She remembers the happy times
she spent in the log cabin with Bill.

Ada has recovered the use of her limbs.
Unfortunately, during the wedding
a child is suffocated by a bouquet
carelessly tossed into its cot.

Hubert's mother has been kidnapped again.
Perhaps Doris will change her mind
at the last moment? Agatha, of course, hopes not . . .

John Ash

Strongman

A strongman you say.
Home from work would stretch his arms
and hang his five sons from them
turning like a roundabout.
A carpenter who could punch nails
into wood with a clenched fist,
chest like a barrel with a neck
that was like holding onto a tree.

In the final hour
your hands between the sheets
to lift him to the lavatory
slipped under a frame of bones like plywood.
No trouble – he said. No trouble, Dad –
you said. And he died in the cradle of your arms.

Tony Curtis

Everybody's Mother

Of course
everybody's mother always and
so on . . .

Always never
loved you enough
or too smothering much.

Of course you were the Only One, your
mother
a machine
that shat out siblings, listen

everybody's mother
was the original Frigid-
aire Icequeen clunking out
the hardstuff in nuggets, mirror-
slivers and ice-splinters that'd stick
in your heart.

Absolutely everyone's mother
was artistic when she was young.

Everyone's mother
was a perfumed presence with pearls, remote
white shoulders when she
bent over in her ball dress
to kiss you in your crib.

Everybody's mother slept with the butcher
for sausages to stuff you with.

Everyone's mother
mythologised herself. You got mixed up
between dragon's teeth and blackmarket stockings.

Naturally
she failed to give you
Positive Feelings
about your own sorry
sprouting body (it was a bloody shame)

but she did
sit up all night sewing sequins
on your carnival costume

so you would have a good time

and she spat
on the corner of her hanky and scraped
at your mouth with sour lace till you squirmed

so you would look smart

And where
was your father all this time?
Away
at the war, or
in his office, or any-
way conspicuous for his
Absence, so

what if your mother did
float around above you
big as a barrage balloon
blocking out the light?

Nobody's mother can't not never do nothing right.

Liz Lochhead

A Birthday Poem
for Rachael

For every year of life we light
a candle on your cake
to mark the simple sort of progress
anyone can make,
and then, to test your nerve or give
a proper view of death,
you're asked to blow each light, each year,
out with your own breath.

James Simmons

Birthdays

When I was six
Everyone had birthday parties.
We always had Dead Lions,
Musical Bumps, Being Sick
And Pass the Parcel . . .

Between each wrapper
Round the swollen present
Lay tucked a toffee
Or a lollipop –
And everybody got a turn
At taking off a layer.

When I was nine, I learned
That the way the music stopped
Was not by chance:
My father's gaze took in
Each trembling lip, each face,
Each pair of hopeful eyes.

When I was twelve, I realised
With some surprise
That later on in life
There's no one there
To press the switch
And make sure
That everything is fair
And everybody
Gets their
Share.

Trevor Millum

Grans

I loved me gran,
Me dad's mam,
She was different from me mam's mam,
Me other gran,
She always baked cake with currants in,
Her hands messy with flour,
She wiped on her pinny,
Before she sipped her Guinness,
And gave me some,
She had a budgie,
Always sitting on the sideboard mirror,
Droppings dropping into a saucer ashtray.
Just missing the only photo of me grandad,
With his cap on the side of his head,
I used confetti once,
To try and clean it,
But it bit me finger
Still I loved me gran's budgie,
And I loved me gran even more,
That's me dad's mam,
But, me mam's mam,
Me other gran,
She chased me with a poker,
And shouted and swore at me,
But that must have been,
Because I was cheeky,
She had a dog called
"Where are yer?"
It was looked after better than me,
She'd put its dinner out, and shout,
"Where are yer?"

And this dog would come from nowhere,
I stood on its paw once,
It bit me,
And left a tooth in me leg,
I cried,
I had to have a needle,
I cried again,
I went back to kick it,
But I didn't
It might have left all its teeth in me,
But I did throw stones at it,
She never had a photo of me other grandad,
I never saw him,
Maybe she chased him with a poker.

Chris Darwin

Grandma and the Blitz

My grandma sat on the bed,
spilling over the edge
like a huge lump of dough.
Her eyes looked already dead,
her mouth dropped long beads of spit
onto her grey nightgown:
one glance and I was off –
sure she was having a fit.
I was only ten, and wrong
about a lot of things:
who Mr Chamberlain
was, why Germans yelled "Achtung!"
how many guns the Spitfire
carried inside each wing;
but I was nearly right
about grandma – the doctor
said she had suffered a stroke.
My mother sent me out
to play, and for three days
hardly bothered me or spoke.
I was glad to be alone –
those were exciting times,
with bombers on their way
and most of the children gone
from the city to seaside
and country. There were air-
raid shelters to explore,
barrage balloons overhead,
a strange anti-aircraft gun
under camouflage nets
in the park, and no school

to interfere with my fun.
Some time after grandma died
the children drifted back
and the city was blitzed.
"Thank goodness your grandma's dead,"
my mother sighed one cold night,
as we crouched in the dark
of the cellar with bombs
exploding to left and right,
"This would have killed her." The past
didn't interest me;
I was impatient for
the "All Clear," and then breakfast,
and then the morning treats:
swastika-marked tail-fins,
and shrapnel and shell shards
picked from the smoking wet streets.

Tony Connor

Granny's Tale

'Your granny had a dreadful flight.
And that is why her hair is white.
And that is why she don't speak right.

'I shuddud in the glavering gloom
as homing through the only wood
I skibbed and teetered past Tog's tomb.

'The path went skinny by a brook
where heaved an owly-headed tree
and on its mozzy trunk a hook.

'There Tog the Ribber once had dingled
while jags and maggies pigged his bones
and where they dropped he rose and wingled.

'His shrieklich ghost and howling bones
had driven men crazy far and wild;
and I all sibble on my lones,

'must pass where Tog had done men dread.
I tibtoed priggled all with fear,
then heard a twittling overhead.

'It was no owl or roasting dook.
It was no friendly joking dad,
but Tog there dingling on his hook.

'I shrikked, 'Oh woly, woly me!'
as Tog begun to clumber down,
unhooking arm and leg and knee.

'He did, but then his black-bone hitched.
I heard him swore. He could not move,
but as he rootled, tugged and twitched,

'I rin. I never rin nor faster;
my liddle fleet went like the wind,
as Tog hobbed clitter clotter after.

'And still he come. I heard his snork.
He snorked green breath upon my nick.
I rin. I rin. He seemed to walk.

'But still he come. I felt his titch.
His shankle tried to trib me up.
But then I reached the fozzle ditch.

'Oh highly, highly fozzle ditch!
Most blost of all the highly high!
He could not pass. He guv a skritch.

'And as I twiddled round to look,
I saw Tog's grozzly heap of bones
go staggering back towards their hook.

'Home, home! My mam a tear she shed.
My daddling kussed his liddle girl
and popped me in my cosly bed.

'But ever since on owly nights
if I should hear the grunting wind,
I have to sleep all round with lights.

'And that is why gran fears the night.
And that is why her hair is white.
And that is why she don't speak right.'

Paul Coltman

All Your Night

Squeeze me, Daddy
squeeze me with all your night.

Save me from dumb dream horrors
that heckle in the not-still hours,
that beat like rain in a blizzard
on my black-filled window
in the dead of dark.

Keep me from the shifting phantoms
that grin shiny in my dream forests,
kill the ogres without pity
that clamour and bang at the door,
stop the beasts in black cupboards
that quarrel and scream red rage
and the mad cats whose scratching claws rip
the paper peace of my dreams.

Closely fold me in your father touch;
far from fear keep me safe
wrapped in the quilts of your comfort.

Stop my night mares from galloping,
their thudding is waking me up;
put them in sleep paddocks
or tell them to graze on the green.

Hold me in the comfort-filled warm
of your tight strong arms
so behind my clenched eyes
only the good dreams come.

Cliff Yates   92

Coming to Terms

The man and the boy worked
together all Sunday afternoon.
They soaped and they squeezed,
lathering the grimy paintwork,
lacing the street with foam.
They talked in a comfortable
'Pass the sponge, please,' kind of
way as they scoured and scrubbed
in the sun. The boy wrote his
name in soapsuds on the bonnet.

He looked up at the man. 'I
expect your mummy's dead by now,'
he said. The man nodded, surprised.
'Well,' the child said, 'I expect
she was very old.' The man thought
about how permanent his mother
had been when he was five. He
remembered her young smell, her
rounded arms. He sighed. And
they went on washing the car.

Moira Andrew

Forbidden Games

A lifetime, and I see them still:
My aunt, my mother, silently
Held by the stove's unflinching eye
Inside the tall house scaled with slate.
The paper boy runs up the hill,
Cries *'Echo!'* to the black-blown sky.
The tin clock on the kitchen shelf
Taps seven. And I am seven. And lie
Flat on the floor playing a game
Of *Snakes & Ladders* by myself.

Upstairs, my father in his bed,
Shadowed still by the German War,
A thin light burning at his head,
To me is no more than a name
That's also mine. I wonder what
The two women are waiting for.
My aunt puts down her library book.
My mother winds a bit of wool.
Each gives to each a blinded look.
'Your father's with the angels now.'
Which of them speaks I cannot tell.
And then I say to them, 'I know.'
And give the dice another throw.

Charles Causley

View from a Bus

Women chicken strut
across wasteland
trying to avoid wet feet
open toed sandals snuggle
into damp grass
scarves cling to curls
carefully pinned to heads
bent on tonight's dance

Louise Hudson

Women on a Seaside Postcard, 1914

In huge hats and hobble skirts
You have stopped to chat on the Rock Walk.
Sun touches your white sleeves, the tidy path,
Cactus, hydrangea-shrubs and palms, the famous rocks.
The length of your gentle shadows suggests
It is late afternoon.

One of you holds a toy dog on a leash.
One of you moves – an arm is out of focus.
You gossip for ever in your absurd
Hats, not an umbrella between you. Don't you know
Across the water the weather has broken?
It will break here soon.

Georgina Hammick

Beauty

Beauty
is a fat black woman
walking the fields
pressing a breezed
hibiscus
to her cheek
while the sun lights up
her feet

Beauty
is a fat black woman
riding the waves
drifting in happy oblivion
while the sea turns back
to hug her shape

Grace Nichols

'In This City . . .'

In this city, perhaps a street.
In this street, perhaps a house.
In this house, perhaps a room.
And in this room a woman sitting,
Sitting in the darkness, sitting and crying
For someone who has just gone through the door
And who has just switched off the light
Forgetting she was there.

Alan Brownjohn

The Hands

To the chopping-block, on which the farmer Sebastian split
logs against the Asturian cold,
the Guardia Civil would shove him and spit:
Now clench the fist with which you made so bold.

Four of them held him under.
He writhed and whimpered, in a state of shock.
The axe would fall, and sunder
the hands that had quarried rock.

With bloody stumps he loped across the land.
They laughed as they shot after him. And when he blared
one came over to stop his mouth with loam.

He lay dead in the field. But his far-fetched hands
would stir at night, and the villagers heard
the fists come blattering on their windows, looking for
    home.

after the German of Erich Arendt

Paul Muldoon

The Migrant from England

A rusty sign and tire tracks
E – Z OFF   E – Z ON

He has a limp now and a scar
and his teeth are plugged.

What do you do where nothing grows,
sell cigarettes?

Nope. Beer and whiskey
if your money's good
just beer and whiskey.

When my wife left
I had just my two sons –
my gospel children.

One of them walked out
when he was sixteen
– never a word –
and came back
six years later.
Hullo Dad he said
. . . I threw him out.

The other still lives
to the north of here
and calls on holidays.
He has no sons and no wife.

I knew a man once who'd say

Praise the Lord who will help Man
Make a Paradise of this Earth!

'It's possible, you know,' he used to say,
'it's possible.'

When death shall close mine eyes.

I saw a book in a store once
a picture of an old Indian in it
left by all his tribe in a cave
or some hole in the rock.

I'm no Indian
shouldn't have to end up that way
in this shack, a filling station,
or any other damn place.

In deserts, they say the Sun is Hell
and the Moon is Paradise,
and that's the way I've found it.

That sign lights up at night for Rheingold
and it's more than a rush candle to me
coming back from a piss in the dark.

I'm looking westward
'cause that's where the sun sets
Down and a-cries to hisself.

Jeffery Wainwright

101

I Used to Hate Andrew Lloyd Webber

I used to hate Andrew Lloyd Webber
But I'm all right now

I had electro convulsive therapy
And it made me see things differently

I went on Wednesdays
Or was it Thursdays
I don't remember which

The doctor asked the question
And the nurse pressed the switch

You book the tickets
Over the phone
And then pick them up
On your way home

I used to write poetry too
Mainly out of spite
But I've stopped doing that now of course
Now that I'm all right

Clive Benson

Moose Malloy's First Poem

Unshaven after a lousy night
this poem hunches its collar,
drives away a Packard sedan
as sharp as a snapped-down hat brim.

Slow feet tap out after dark,
the poem leans back into the shadow
scans the street corner, sticks
a tight smile on the subway.

It's no fool my lovely
with your hair like Van Gogh
had a fire in his palette.

Last night it got scrawled
all over the wall of a cheap hotel
some downtown dive
that rhymed in blue neon.

Today, printed backwards
on the frosted glass of an office door,
the poem's seams bulge at the shoulders

so tell me,
what is its name doing
inside your mouth?

David Harmer

Social Poem

There was a shoe in the road this morning.
A single shoe, and a good one.
No one in it, and the rain pouring down,
but still the shoe stood there,
like a monument to a foot that had passed on.
I should have picked it up,
but it wasn't my size, and what's the use
of a single shoe anyway?
It had gone when I got back. Oh God, what
happens to discarded single shoes?

Jim Burns

A Healthy Meal

The gourmet tastes the secret dreams of cows
tossed lightly in garlic. Behind the greendoor, swish
of oxtails languish on an earthen dish. Here are
wishbones and pinkies; fingerbowls will absolve guilt.

Capped teeth chatter to a kidney or at the breast
of something which once flew. These hearts knew
no love and on their beds of saffron rice they lie
beyond reproach. What is the claret like? Blood.

On table six, the language of tongues is braised
in armagnac. The woman chewing suckling pig
must sleep with her husband later. Leg,
saddle and breast bleat against pure white cloth.

Alter *calf* to *veal* in four attempts. This is
the power of words; knife, tripe, lights, charcuterie.
A fat man orders his *rare* and a fine sweat
bastes his face. There are napkins to wipe the
        evidence

and sauces to gag the groans of abbattoirs. The menu
lists the recent dead in French, from which they order
offal, poultry, fish. Meat flops in the jowls. Belch.
Death moves in the bowels. You are what you eat.

Carol Ann Duffy

Cold Knap Lake

We once watched a crowd
pull a drowned child from the lake.
Blue-lipped and dressed in water's long green silk
she lay for dead.

Then kneeling on the earth,
a heroine, her red head bowed,
her wartime cotton frock soaked,
my mother gave a stranger's child her breath.
The crowd stood silent,
drawn by the dread of it.

The child breathed, bleating
and rosy in my mother's hands.
My father took her home to a poor house
and watched her thrashed for almost drowning.

Was I there?
Or is that troubled surface something else
shadowy under the dipped fingers of willows
where satiny mud blooms in cloudiness
after the treading, heavy webs of swans
as their wings beat and whistle on the air?

All lost things lie under closing water
in that lake with the poor man's daughter.

Gillian Clarke

Wittgenstein on Egdon Heath

the world is everything that is the case
the world is   verythin   ha
the world is eve   in   a   case
the world is   the case
the world is   that   case
the world is   th   is   case
the world is every   case
    world is   hat   case
    world is   hat
    world is   case
    world is   thing
    world is   that
    world is   th   is
    world is   the   se
the world is everything that is the   se
 he   is   the   se
 he   is   th   is
 he   is   that
 he   is eve
 he   is everything
the wor d is everything
the wor d is everything that is the case
 h   o ld   everything
the wo ld is everything that is the case

The first line is a quotation from Wittgenstein's
'Tractatus Logico-Philosophicus'.

Edwin Morgan

Commentary

Someone once said: "I can't write poems about trees or flowers, because I'm not a tree or a flower. I'm a person. I write about people." Fair enough, and I've always used that as a good excuse not to write any nature poetry, but it makes me ask another question: "Do you always have to write as yourself?" In other words, is the 'I' in a poem always the poet, or can a man write as a woman or vice versa? I know that Terry Caffrey isn't a ship welder's mate but he writes about the 'Scouse Apache' as though he knows him well. Duncan Curry is a teacher, and he writes 'McCoy's Last Stand' with an insight that only teachers and desks can have (but desks don't write poems!). Do you think the bit of backwards-writing towards the end of the poem works? Imagine the 'Scouse Apache' meeting the teacher from 'McCoy's Last Stand' in a pub. Perhaps "The Dirty Man" from Stanley Cook's poem could join them?

Sometimes poems can just suggest characters rather than creating fully rounded ones. John Ash does this in his poem 'A Novel', perhaps you could write a review of the novel, or a first chapter? I first saw 'A Novel' right at the bottom of a page in a magazine, and I turned the page to see what came next. I assumed there was another verse. I think that's one of the signs of a good poem, it leaves you wanting more.

Families are fertile ground for poems. Poets are always writing about their parents, grandparents, children, grandchildren, wives, husbands, etc. It might be a good exercise to write a poem about someone in your family and to substitute a silly word for the name of the family member. So, instead of Grandma you put "bullwhip" or "saddlebag". Try it. You'll be amazed. Liz Lochhead ('Everybody's Mother') and Tony Curtis ('Strongman') look at parents in different ways, both avoiding sentimentality, although Tony Curtis only just avoids it.

I like the James Simmon's poem 'A Birthday Poem' even though it rhymes. I'm not that keen on rhymes for rhyme's sake. Sometimes it can really spoil a poem and make your ears ache. It's all a matter of give and take. Sometimes you might as well throw the poem in a nearby lake.

I like Trevor Millum's poem 'Birthdays', because I wish I'd written it myself, simple as that. I'm sure that the phrase "All your night" in Cliff Yates' poem is a child trying to say "All your might". It's a wonderfully dark phrase: let me squeeze you with all my night. It's worth listening out for the things children say.

The three grandma poems that follow are meant to show the different ways that poets can look at the fairly clichéd idea of grandmothers. They all work in their different ways, but my favourite is the Paul Coltman poem 'Granny's Tale', because of the way the strange language takes over and yet the story still carries us along. I love invented languages. Gort nopsock!

Moira Andrew's poem 'Coming to Terms' is a bit like Cliff Yates' 'All Your Night': both look at age from a child's perspective. It's worth having a go at writing as though you're a child, although you should be careful: it can fail horribly.

Charles Causley is a wonderful poet who writes with a brilliant eye for detail: look at the reference to "echo" in line six of 'Forbidden Games'. Death is a big subject and lots of poems have been written about it, but this is one of the best I've read recently.

Following the views of Grandmas and death, there are some views of women. Louise Hudson uses the 'looking from a bus' technique, which can be a useful method of writing poems. I was once on a bus and I saw a man on a golf course let go of his club just after he'd swung it and it landed on the head of another man. This happened in Burton on Trent. I was going to write a poem about it, but I never did. Perhaps you could?

The women in the Georgina Hammick poem 'Women on a Seaside Postcard, 1914' contrast wonderfully with the woman in the Grace Nichols poem 'Beauty'. It's just a question of style, isn't it? Perhaps you could try rewriting these two poems in the style of the other one? 'In This City' is a poem about the loss of love that isn't as tear-stained as these kinds of poems often are. Try and write a serious limerick about the loss of love.

One of the reasons I put 'The Hands' by Paul Muldoon in the book is that it's a sonnet and you have to have at least one sonnet in every poetry anthology or you get fourteen knocks on your door late at night from the sonnet police. I also put it in the book because I found it heart-stoppingly powerful the first time I read it in a magazine, and being the editor of an anthology gives you a marvellous opportunity to put poems you love in front of a wider audience. I'm sure that editors who write in their introductions, "These poems are the most important poems of the twentieth century" really mean, "Here are some poems that I like and some poems by my friends", which is all very well as long as everybody gets the chance to edit at least one anthology.

The Jeffery Wainwright poem 'The Migrant from England' has haunted me for years. Bits of it pop into my head when I'm lying awake at 4am thinking about the world situation. It's a difficult poem, and I don't want to help you with it too much, but it seems to be partly about how loneliness can eventually even seep into the language you use and the way you use it. Now that's profound.

'I Used to Hate Andrew Lloyd Webber' makes me laugh, and I know (going back in a clever way to the theme at the start of these notes) that the "I" in the poem isn't the author. In 'Moose Malloy's First Poem', David Harmer writes as though the poem itself were the gangster; perhaps you could write Tarzan's First Poem, The Gas Fire's First Poem, The Goldfish's First Poem?

I put the 'Social Poem' by Jim Burns in the book because I was once on Stockport station late at night and I saw a train driver holding up one big green shoe. A few days later I read the Jim Burns poem and I carried it about with me for weeks in case I saw the train driver again. Perhaps he'll read this book.

There isn't much to say about the Carol Ann Duffy and Gillian Clarke poems; I put them in because they both nudge us towards compassion in different ways. They make us think, if that's not too simplistic.

The Edwin Morgan poem 'Wittgenstein on Egdon Heath' opens up all kinds of possibilities, which is what poetry in general, and this book in particular, should do. It's a simple technique really, just get a sentence and block out words or letters to form lines of poetry. Have a go. See you after the next section.

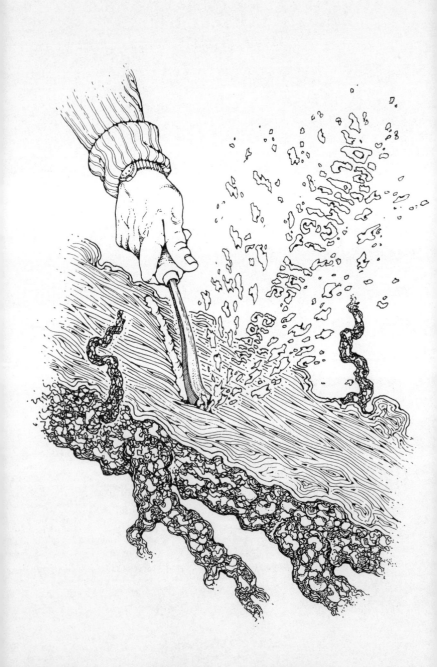

SECTION FOUR:

Against the Grain

Introduction

Introduction

One of the wonderful things about poems is that like fingerprints, clouds and bits of navel fluff, they're all unique. A workshop exercise I often do is to get each member of a group to write a poem using the same title; often they come up with widely different interpretations of the title.

This is more or less what I've done here: I wrote to a number of writers and asked them to write me a poem called 'Against the Grain', with no guidelines as to length and style. The results, as you'll see, are an exciting mixture of styles and approaches.

Arthur Kirby for example, was a member of a writers group I ran with Martyn Wiley at Age Concern in Leicester during 1988. I gave them the title "Against the Grain" as a piece of homework.

Of course it goes without saying that the next stage is for you to write a poem called 'Against the Grain.' It goes without saying so I won't say it.

Against the Grain – Draft

He has grown weary of all the struggle
He can find no peace as he curls up tight
Like a foetus on a mattress of thorns

He is being punished by their jungle laws
Finds no escape from the scratching claws
Of those who never seem to leave his side

Yet he knows about love, it crept up to him
Brought unexpected sunshine to his cold room
Brushed away the cobwebs and the crawling fears

Then kissed his fevered brow and brought relief
Breathed life into a corpse with magic words
She had wanted no reward but his slow smile

He had to learn to live without her close to him
She had tried to cry his tears and feel his hurt
Now he must learn to carry his own heavy chains

For the loving care had taken all her strength
She is resting now, there among the flowers
And he is not allowed to even keep them watered

He sees only the eyes of hate around him now
The message round his cell walls cuts him deep
"Black scum", daubed there by his white masters

Arthur Kirby

Against the Grain

He has grown weary
Of all the struggle
He can find no peace
Curled up like a foetus
On a mattress of thorns

He is being punished
By their jungle laws
And may never escape
The scratching claws
Of those around him

Yet he knows about love
It crept into his room
Kissed his fevered brow
She really tried too hard
For one who was so frail

She wept her last tear
And now he must learn
To lift his own chains
And let her tired body
Sleep among the flowers

He stares around him
All he sees now is hate
It is written on the walls
Of his damp, dark cell
By all the white masters.

Arthur Kirby

Writing the Poem

Ian has got me up a gum-tree with today's
homework 'Against the Grain', it has so many
different interpretations. I thought about consulting
my dictionary to see just how many interpretations
it has, but then I watched a documentary on
Channel Four about apartheid. I thought about all
the people who are never allowed to live complete
lives, either through poverty, bigotry, illness or
whatever, then the figure of Nelson Mandela
flashed on my sight-screen and 'Against the Grain'
was no longer a problem piece of homework.

Arthur Kirkby

Against the Grain – Draft

The jack-plane jarred, bucked
And stuck;
I'd gone against the grain,
Despite all he'd said.
I pulled it free and looked where the blade
Had ripped up against the rings of oak.

The circular saw whined and snarled
A wild dog penned in the corner,
Where my father stood, dividing up
Planks through the long rhythm of the day.

The coke stove burned, acrid,
Until I piled in wood shavings
And the sweet pine-smoke came;
Birds' feet skittered on the thin roof;
In winter he'd rescue them, half-starved
And warm them in that sullen heat.

I was building my first guitar,
Not wanting to be told
Which way the grain ran;
It all ran against his:
BB King and Howlin' Wolf versus Chopin and Liszt.

I'd hear him playing on a Sunday night, cooing
Through the floor where he sat at the Broadwood,
But filtering into late night R & B:
Wild guitars soaring through my sleep,
Chopin and Liszt soothing his.

But we finished it together, fretted,
Varnished, strings tightened to pitch;
Plugged into the record player,
And the first chords of the blues
Rising through the house like birds.

Graham Mort

Against the Grain

The jack-plane jarred and stuck:
I'd gone against the grain,
Despite all he'd said –
I looked where steel
Should have smoothed the edge:
It had ripped against growth-rings instead.

Penned in the corner, my father stood,
The circular saw whined then snarled,
Sawing up plank after plank,
Measuring the days in lengths of wood.

The coke stove burned acrid,
Until I piled in wood-shavings
And sweet pine-smoke came;
Birds' feet skittered on the tar roof –
In winter he'd rescue them, half-starved
And warm them with the sullen flame.

I was building my first guitar,
Not wanting to be told
Which way the grain went;
It all ran against his:
BB King versus Chopin and Liszt,
The outcry against the lament.

The piano cooing through late R & B,
I'd hear him playing on a Sunday night;
Gentle waltzes soothed his sleep,
Electrified solos soared through me.

We finished it together, fretted,
Plugged into the amplifier,
Strings tightened to pitch;
The fumbled first chords rose like birds:
I saw his blue-veined hands let them pass,
But tense and grip the air and twitch.

Graham Mort

Writing the Poem

*When I was asked to write a poem with the title
'Against the Grain' my imagination immediately
returned to my father's carpentry workshop. I spent
my early years there, playing amongst shavings and
sawdust, hammering pieces of wood together and
feeding off-cuts to the coke stove: thirty years on, I
can still smell that as if it was burning under my
nose now.*

*Years later, I turned on the radio one Saturday
afternoon to discover the first musical love of my
life: Mike Raven's Rhythm & Blues programme.
Too hard-up to buy one, I set about making my first
electric guitar. My father treated the whole affair
with the utmost suspicion, but the final effort was a
collaboration – and it worked! My father still
doesn't like the blues and jazz I listen to, but he's
happy that I'm involved in playing music in my
own way.*

*What I learned most of all was that you can't
force the wood to behave as you want it to. It's got a
life and tenacity of its own, which you have to
respect when you're working it. My father learned
the same thing about his son: he ended up by
respecting my determination, recognising the same
stubborn grain that ran through his own character.*

*Later still, when I began to write my first poems I
realised that the same thing was happening there.
The poems emerged from my pen almost in one
piece, and although I could chamfer and smooth
them here and there, it was impossible to reshape*

them completely, to go against their intrinsic grain.
They had come through me, like radio waves
through a receiver, and I could never own them: like
the music, they belonged to anyone who would
listen.

Graham Mort

Against the Grain – Draft

I could be anywhere as window-framed
I watch the sky. Sometimes it is blue
as dreams or white as sleep or maybe mourning
(for white is sorrow. The pretty women in their
    bright saris
told me that. They are pent up now, like me,
behind the gloss of wooden doors).
Only the birds are at home here; patterns of wings
and vertigo against the sky. I don't look down.
I feel there is a suction where the women
tick along the veins of path across the grass
towards the shops, behind their crippled prams.

Paint on walls dispossesses – NIGGERS
GO HOME WOGS OUT drives me upwards.
Night binds us all. I think the tower must turn
into a pinnacle of light, all those eyes,
unblinking, on a carnival of breaking glass,
a quick heartbeat of voices. My window squares
to black. I wait for the lift's exhalation,
and the squeak of soft-soled trainers by the
    door,
for the first blow of the axe, splintering
my peace, my life, my home.

Shirley Bell

126

Against the Grain

I could be anywhere as window-framed
I watch the sky. Sometimes it is blue
as dreams, then white as sleep or maybe mourning
(for white is sorrow. Pretty women in bright saris
told me that. They are pent up now, like me,
behind the gloss of wooden doors).
Only birds are at home here: patterns of wings
and vertigo against the sky. I don't look down.
I feel there is a suction where mothers tick
behind their crippled prams on veins
of path.

Darkness walls us in. Outside, the tower
must turn into a pinnacle of light;
all those eyes, unblinking, on a carnival
of breaking glass. My window squares to black.
And every night – since paint on walls
(NIGGERS GO HOME) unsettled me – I wait
for the exhalation of the lift, that quick
heartbeat of voices, and a squeal
of soft-soled trainers at my door.
Wait for the first blow, splintering
my life.

Shirley Bell

*Nothing seems more against the grain than the way
people were environmentally 'designed' to live in a
home suspended in a monolithic tower block. When
I was seventeen, I had a boyfriend who lived on the
top floor of a tower block in Birmingham; I found
visiting him so vertigo-producing that our affair
was much briefer than it might have been! To me,
against the grain also means living unnaturally in a
non-physical way – growing into the wrong shape
spiritually or ethically, or being forced into a
deforming way of life through outside pressures.*

*These two ideas, then, gave me the location of the
poem and the situation of the people in it. Everyone
and everything is against the grain – the people
whose 'home' is no such thing, even without the
pressures which imprison them, and the unnatural
behaviour of their persecutors, who are also victims
of the way they live.*

*I hope the changes between the Draft and final
versions give some pointers to my working methods.
The ideas were there in their entirety before I wrote
a word: from then on it was a battle to express them
as clearly and economically as I could. Although I
didn't want a poem which depended heavily on the
imagery of wood – smooth, polished, strokeable
surfaces with the grain, contrasting with damaged,
splintering, unworkable surfaces against the grain –
I thought it was important to have a literal
counterpoint to the metaphorical use of the title.*

Therefore, I felt I was justified in introducing
"wooden doors" in the first stanza and "splintering"
in the second.

Shirley Bell

Against the Grain   *[handwritten: DRAFT 3]*

[handwritten: lane]
[handwritten struck: Pakiw]
green ~~centre~~ national park

grey silence   horizontal rain

[handwritten: Wrecked?]
[handwritten struck: Suddenly] knocked sideways ~~suddenly~~ *[handwritten: ← stet]*

[handwritten: Sound of] hover mower, kitchen whisk,

[handwritten arrow] metal whirling wrecked roaring

[handwritten arrow] motor mountain bike ~~mud metal~~

[handwritten: mud] rider mounted like a mantis

Dear Mr Finch,

While appreciating your concern

we have to point out ~~that~~

public access prime consideration

legitimate environmental

motorcycular 14 meter gash

existing tracks a/nimber under

sub section 23 (A) adopted

formal vehicular route hard

luck

[handwritten: individual] *[scribble]* *[handwritten: the deeply offensive menace —]*
~~intrusive~~ action against ~~individual menace~~

I am spoking to win but

I am sparking to wine bit

I have spungled two woan bites

I hill sponking the wild bits

I half speech ningto wally but

I have sproking two three *[handwritten: bo]*

I have speaking to four but

I have speaking toe fun

130

I am spoken abundant

I have spoken to one

but

~~but~~

I am isolated by inferior strength

I am unable because my sight

I cannot since religion

I am full of moral persuasion

~~I am too quick Jiffer~~ ←

I lack focus I am advancing in age

Kawasaki can cross country at 80 mph

which
~~There are many~~ solution**s** ?

~~I can't shape this~~
~~I can change nothing~~

I can do nothing but talk,
~~I am quick~~   wave my arms
~~I~~

    tin tacks

    wire

    money

    deafness

    afforestation

    lions

one ?
Which ~~is best?~~ ~~change the grain?~~

You decide.

March 1989

131

Against the Grain

green lane   national park
grey silence   horizontal rain
knocked sideways suddenly
sound of hover mower, kitchen
whisk metal whirling wrecked
roaring motor mountain bike
mud rider mounted like a mantis

> Dear Mr Finch,
> While appreciating your concern
> we have to point out
> public access prime consideration
> legitimate environmental
> motorcycular 14 meter
> gash existing tracks a number under
> sub section 23 (A) adopted
> formal vehicular route hard
> luck.

individual action against the deeply offensive menace –

I am spoking to win but
I em sparking to wine bit
I have spungled two woan bites
I hill sponking the wild bits

I half speech ningto wally but
I have sproking two three bo
I have speaking to four but
I have speaking toe fun

I am spoken abundant
I have spoken to one
                    but

I am isolated by inferior strength
I an unable because my sight
I cannot since religion
I am full of moral persuasion
I can do nothing but talk
wave my arms   advance in age

Kawasaki can cross country at 80 mph

Which solution?

        tin tacks
        money
        deafness
        afforestation

        lions

You decide.

Peter Finch

Writing the Poem

*Opposing forces confront each other in the
countryside. The walker meets the helmeted
motorbike rider. Arbitration by a third party is
inconclusive. What can be done? Talk about it,
suffer the inevitable communications problems, live
with the problem until the generations change. The
poem presupposes a conflict of values between
youth and middle age. It offers surreal solutions.
How do you prevent one person's enjoyment from
becoming the bane of another's? Bribe them, break
them, ignore them, plant trees to stop them. The
piece is an analogy for conflicts on a larger stage.
This is my land and I will march in it. Try to stop
me. You can't. I have used a number of methods –
permutation of the phrase "I have spoken to one
but" to lead the reader through the varieties of
possible misunderstandings; adapted found material
in the letter to reflect the effectiveness of our
institutions; a touch of surrealism to show the way
out. It is a performance piece, of course, meant for
shouting. Who is rubbing against whose grain? You
decide.*

Peter Finch

Against the Grain

Someone must count the bodies that come up
one by one out of the fire, up from
the gloomy cradle of the North Sea
that has weighted and washed them, months.

Someone must number them, name each one
by the fingerprints, by the rings, by the teeth,
someone must stare at the remnants of the dead
from Zeebrugge, Kings Cross, Piper Alpha:

more oil there than under all Arabia,
I recall long ago, that we bought and paid for.
We're dying of neglect. My country
is a free enterprise disaster zone.

And now someone must count them all: one, one.
Someone must zip them into a bag
and bury them, tally the ongoing total,
put up a stone. It goes against the grain.

Ken Smith

Writing the Poem

*Well, I may have salvaged some of this, after having
struggled and given up on it. Initially I decided that
writing a poem about disasters was itself against the
grain. Going back to it some weeks after I'd
abandoned it, I saw there were things I could get rid
of. In effect these were two stanzas in which I'd
become too overt in saying that the reason for all
these disasters is the greed of the rich, backed by the
government, in cut corners and an eye to safety
regulations, in failed maintenance on the tubes and
railways, ferries and oil platforms. You don't see
these two missing stanzas because I'm embarrassed
by them; they're weak and are where the poem
went wrong. All I have to do is press 'Delete' and
they've gone back into the electricity supply.*

    *External events also had their effect in
abandoning the poem: the Lockerbie plane disaster,
quickly followed by another plane crash on the M1
put me off my appetite for disasters, and since then
the trains keep colliding, and certainly the first of
these couldn't be blamed on the government. So the
poem collapsed under its own weight. Sometimes I
think it's a good thing to abandon it, walk away
from it, saying what does it matter whether I ever
write this or not?*

    *I saw then that what I was left with was almost
good enough. Ideally, I need more time, but this
must go as it is to the waiting printer. Deadlines are
useful too. They focus the mind. As it is, the poem is
close to my original intention, for I see from my*

notebook a handwritten page that begins:

> <u>Looking at Bodies</u>
> *They come up, one by one,*
> *out of the fire, up from*
> *the unlit dark at the bottom*
> *of the North Sea to be counted.*

From the notebook I would have worked straight
into this machine, erasing each draft as it changed,
so there are no worksheets. The difference between
the initial notebook entry and the final version of it
is the result of polishing like a stone in water. I think
where I was stuck was in being given a commission,
in part. Maybe it's a bit like being in school and
given a theme. It's only worse if you're not given a
theme. I felt I had to say something, when in fact
I'm under no obligation to say anything at all.

That's all.

Ken Smith

Against the Grain – Draft

Against the Grain

"Simon," said Miss Gray one day,
"Now you're a dreamy groovy guy.
Would you take part in our school play?"
And she was giving me the eye.

"Up on a stage, and that, I says.
I mean that's sump-in new for me.
I don't do much unless it pays."
"Ah, but I'm sure you will agree."

And she torched me with those lovely glims.
I really fancied her, you see.
She was one of these magic dames.
I reckoned that the least I'd be

would be James Bond with those glam blondes
all of them looking like Miss Gray
swanning about and saying, "Bond.
I go for you in a big way."

But what it was was a crappy play
called A MIDSUMMER-NIGHT'S DREAM
and there was no one like Miss Gray
but creepy Greeks who got up steam

wandering about in this freaky wood
where there was fairies, stuff like that,
prancing about in the nude.
There was drugs and dukes and lots of chat

and gits that was always getting lost
and chasing each other through the night,
and sometimes they would have a doss
and then they'd snog or have a fight.

I learned the poetry they said,
I thought a lot of it was bull.
It gave me a pain in the head.
But Miss Gray thought it was real cool.

"Simon, you were brill," she said.
I bowed and nearly split my jeans.
I really felt a proper ned.
Them Greeks are a bunch of might have beens.

Why didn't they have a map or that?
Why did they go on about the moon?
And who was that old donkey prat,
and that wet twit called 'Oberon'.

"I'll tell you what," I told Miss Gray,
bleeding hypocrite I was,
"I really loved doing that play"
(But I'd far rather have done Jaws.)

It only proves that you can speak
without a clue of what you say,
and that you've got to be a Greek
to speak posh English in a play.

Iain Crichton Smith

Writing the Poem

*This poem caused me great difficulty, partly
because I wished to make the contrast between a
classic play like A Midsummer-Night's Dream and
the language spoken by the boy. One of my
problems was whether I should make the teacher
speak in her own voice. I decided to make her speak
in his voice, the way he would hear her. I chose the
subject because I have always been terrified of
public appearances and I would never ever take
part in a play. I would always have the feeling that
I would forget my words. I wrote the poem in rhyme
because I think you can get better effects in rhyme
than in free verse, with a poem that is meant to be
comic.*

Iain Crichton Smith

The Laughing Warrior: Against the Grain.

Warrior where do you go
When your muscle is clutched by cramp

Warrior where do you rest
That your wounds may heal

Warrior where do you cry
For your mother, the hostage,

Warrior where do you sit,
To catch your racing breath

Warrior you still laugh

Lemn Sissay

Writing the Poem

*In a strange way the laugh of this warrior is as sad
as it is happy, but in its very loudness it defies the
tears to come out, the forehead to frown and the
hands to clasp the head. The laughing warrior
would die laughing and at the last second a twinkle
of sadness would spark in his eye. He is a permanent
source of intrigue to his friends and his enemies. In
this poem I try to hold him still upon the paper for
an exclusive interview. I hope the poem's simplicity
underlines its complexity . . .*

and . . . or . . .

*The laughing warrior. This title came in to my head
after tearing it apart for a poem. For some reason I
found myself thinking about revolutionaries, many
of them were happy. Steve Biko is a prime example
(he died for his cause). The laughing warrior seems
to be as much a child's hero as a world hero. It
conjured up so much that I knew this poem had to
be written. In this poem I try to hold him still on the
paper for an exclusive interview, maybe I am
looking for his answer so I can use it myself. The
poem is a simple series of questions and images
deliberately conjured so as to underline its
complexity. I prefer writing it and reading it, than
explaining it.*

Lemn Sissay

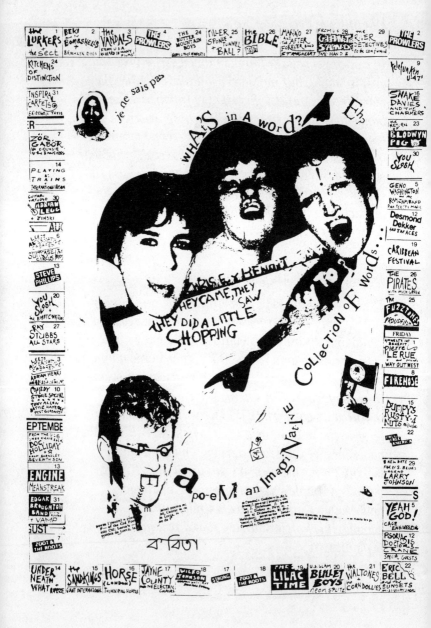

the LURKERS 1 / the sect
BEKI and the BOMBSHELLS 2 / Brooklyn Dogs
the VANDALS 3 / From U.S.A. As heard in many films
THE PROWLERS 4
THE BUTTER MOUNTAIN BOYS 24
KILLER 25 / SPONGE + TUNNEL BALL?
the BIBLE 26
MARIA'O 27 / and After the FOREVER BAND / STRAIGHTHEART
FROM U.S 28 / THE CRAMPS AGAIN
THE TERRIER DETECTIVES 29 / to be confirmin
THE PROWLERS 2

KITCHENS OF DISTINCTION 24

je ne sais pas

WHAtS in A word? Eh?

Telefunken U-47 9

SNAK DAVIES AND THE CHAMPERS 16

We RETURN 23 / BLODWYN PIG! 6

YOU SLOSH 30

INSPIRAL CARPETS 31 / ERIC FULL TAKIS

R

ZOR GABOR 7 / (or siouxsie & the banshees)

PLAYING the TRAINS 14 / INTERNATIONAL RESCUE

Guitar Virtuoso ADRIAN LEGG 30 / + JINSKI

AU

LEEDS ALTERNATIVE CABARET 6 / SUITCASE CIRCUS etc

STEVE PHILLIPS 13

YOU SLOSH 20 + the ROOTIC WRITERS

RAY STUBBS ALL STARS 27

LEEDS ALTERNATIVE CABARET 3 / ADRIAN HENRI ...

COMEDY STORE SPECIAL 10 / + TONY ALLEN / ATTIE HARKIN / POST GLASGOW?

EPTEMBE / FROM THE U.S DOC HOLLIDAY / from Barnsley SEVENTH SON

ENGINE 13 / MEANSTREAK

EDGAR BROUGHTON BAND etc 31 / + VAMP

UST / ZOOT & the ROOTS 7

ARISE, X HENRIT

THEY CAME, THEY SAW / THEY DID A LITTLE SHOPPING

CoLLeCtioN oF words...

GENO WASHINGTON and the RAM JAM BAND 5 / Pan Tetti's music

Desmond Dekker and the ACES 12

CARIBBEAN FESTIVAL 19

THE PIRATES with MICK GREEN 26

the FUZZTONES PROUDFUSE 25

FRIDAY / AMNESTY INT'L BENEFIT / Pierre LE RUE / + WAY OUT WEST 8

FIREHOSE

DUMPY'S RUSTY NUTS 15 / millions

UNCLE SAM AMERICA 22

a po-eM an ImagiNaTive

NEW DATE 29 / FROM U.S. BLUES LEGEND LARRY JOHNSON

S

YEAH! GOD! 5 / CAGE ENGINEERING

PSORIA 12 / DOCTORS 21S CRANE / SPECIAL GUESTS

কবিতা

UNDER NEATH WHAT 14 / Ripple
the SANDKINGS 15 / GIANT INTERNATIONAL
HORSE LONDON 16 / THUNDERING HEARTS
JAYNE COUNTY 17 / the ELECTRIC CHAIRS
WILCO JOHNSON 18
17 STRONG
ZOOT & the ROOTS 18
THE LILAC TIME 19
US GLAM 20 / BULLET BOYS / NEON SPLIT
the WALTONES 21 / with CORN DOLLIES
ERIC BELL 22 / and the SUNSETS

SECTION FIVE

A Summer's Day

yir eyes ur
eh
a mean yir

pirrit this wey
ah a thingk yir
byewtifl like ehm

fact
fact a thingk yir
ach a luvyi thahts

thahts
jist thi wey it iz like
thahts ehm
aw ther iz ti say

Tom Leonard

Love Poem for Janet

Shut up Janet
Just shut up Janet
Janet shut up
Dammit Janet shut up
Janet dammit
Will you shut up
Shut up Janet dammit
Kick the car Janet
Go on kick it dammit
That won't fix it
Janet
The car didn't get us lost dammit
You did Janet
I can get lost on my own dammit
I don't need your help Janet
Oh for god's sake
Shut up Janet dammit
Dammit Janet shut up
Just shut it
Will you just
Shut it dammit Janet
Dammit Janet shut it
Janet dammit
Where are you going Janet?
Dammit Janet
Where are you going?
Oh dammit
One eency weency
Little bit
Of criticism
Janet

And you walked out
Dammit!

Christopher Mills

OK Gimme

OK gimme
OK gimme

Two quarter pounders
Two cheeseburgers
Four side orders
French fries
Two Coca-Colas
Two Doc Peppers
All to go?
Yeah! All to go

We got to go

Over thirty-five million sold
Over thirty-five million sold

OK that will be
Nine dollars and fifty

Have a nice day
Have a nice day
Have a nice day

Martyn Wiley

Trainspotter

Trainspotter trainspotter trainspotter
Train train
Trainspotter trainspotter trainspotter
Train train

He's got the anorak
He's got the duffle bag
He's got the big notebook
And a pocket full of pens
Fountain pens and cartridge pens
And all those flippin' biros

And all those flippin' biros

Derek's ready
Derek's ready
Derek's ready
For the
Red light
Orange light
Green light
GO!
WHOOSH!!
MISSED IT!

Trainspotter trainspotter trainspotter
Train train
Trainspotter trainspotter trainspotter
Train train

He's got the thermos flask
He's got the sandwiches

He's got the big bag of crisps
And a pocket full of sweets
Chocolate bars and Yorkie bars
And all those flippin' Penguins

And all those flippin' Penguins

Derek's ready
Derek's ready
Derek's ready
For the
Red light
Orange light
Green light
GO!
WHOOSH!!
MISSED IT!!

Missed it. Again.

Have another go
Have another go
Get a closer look
Get a closer look
At the
Red light
Orange light
Green light
GO!
WHOOSH!!

Ouch!!
Caught it!!!

Right in the back
Right in the back
Right in the back of the anorak.

So now they're spotting Derek
So now they're spotting Derek

Trainspotter trainspotter trainspotter
Train train
Trainspotter trainspotter trainspotter
Train train

They've got the duffle bag
That's in Crewe
They've got the family pack of crisps
That's in Wick
They've got the big notebook
That's loose leaf –
Covers all the regions

Covers all the regions

Mind you so does Derek
Mind you so does Derek
With his
Red light
Orange light
Green light
GO!
WHOOSH!!

Trainspotter trainspotter trainspotter
Train train
Trainspotter trainspotter trainspotter
Train train
Neeeyaah!!

David Harmer and Martyn Wiley

Country Dancing

Polka
do it
clap a lot
Polka
do it again
those on the edge do it
posh ones do it
arch, sway their legs, swing
others falter
don't do it, won't do it,
can't do it again.
The caller has rubber lips and stiff arms, he goes:
bop she doobie oobie dub dub rapidly rapidly
pairs walled by tight shoes get their roots pulled;
strip the willow down
move all the chairs into the centre
girls turn round, link up with knotted handkerchiefs
    and pass their legs over the men's shoulders
rhythm increases
friends hold each other just in case
backs bent, they make V signs,
most of the men have on flared trousers.
The last part of the dance must be done
speedily because there is very little
time in the music
keep your teeth together
hum, snap your fingers, hum.

Peter Finch

Source: *American Dance Instruction Manual*

The Holy Places

You won't get across to Lindisfarne,
not tonight you won't. Tide's coming in.

> *Our Arthur died when he were nearly ten.*
> *That's when I started going to the Holy Places.*
> *Being a railway man I get free passes.*
> *Put me bike and stuff in the luggage van.*
> *I travel light. Canvas bags I got.*
> *That Marj were a bugger she were, smoked in bed*
> *so I left her, couldn't stand the way she cried*
> *behind her specs. Rome I've seen, the lot.*
> *Walsingham. Moscow with me Union card.*
> *That were alright. Assisi. Been to Lourdes.*
> *I'm not religious, mind. I've touched the Pope.*
> *That place in Ireland, that were bloody good,*
> *everyone on their knees and drinking hard.*
> *Get to that Lindisfarne tonight I hope.*

Not till tomorrow. Tide'll soon be in.
> *Oh – but tomorrow I've got to catch me train.*

Meg Peacock

(Found poem: from a conversation on the road to
Lindisfarne.)

154

(Shades of Gone)

To confuse the Evil Spirits
that surrounded our home
Grandfather would lie down
and pretend to be dead.

Never to rise again.

Never again
to see
the blue green hills
   of home.

Never again
to hear
the voices of children
raised in laughter.

Never again
to witness
the loving hands
   of his wife
sculpting beams of sunlight
as they flicker upon the forest
   ground.

Charlie Mehrhoff

Mr Waterman

'Well now, we're quite private in here. You can tell me your troubles. The pond, I think you said . . .'

'We never really liked that pond in the garden. At times it was choked with a sort of weed, which, if you pulled one thread, gleefully unravelled until you had an empty basin before you and the whole of the pond in a soaking heap at your side. Then at other times it was as clear as gin, and lay in the grass staring upwards. If you came anywhere near, the gaze shifted sideways, and it was you that was being stared at, not the empty sky. If you were so bold as to come right up to the edge, swaggering and talking loudly to show you were not afraid, it presented you with so perfect a reflection that you stayed there spellbound and nearly missed dinner getting to know yourself. It had hypnotic powers.'

'Very well. Then what happened?'

'Near the pond was a small bell hung on a bracket, which the milkman used to ring as he went out to tell us upstairs in the bedroom that we could go down and make the early-morning tea. This bell was near a little avenue of rose-trees. One morning, very early indeed, it tinged loudly and when I looked out I saw that the empty bottles we had put out the night before were full of bright green pondwater. I had to go down and empty them before the milkman arrived. This was only the beginning. One evening I was astounded to find a brace of starfish coupling on the ornamental stone step of the pool, and, looking up, my cry to my wife to come and see was stifled by the sight of

156

a light peppering of barnacles on the stems of the rose-trees. The vermin had evidently crept there, taking advantage of the thin film of moisture on the ground after the recent very wet weather. I dipped a finger into the pond and tasted it: it was brackish.'

'*But it got worse.*'

'It got worse: one night of howling wind and tempestuous rain I heard muffled voices outside shouting in rural tones: "Belay there, you lubbers!" "Box the foresail capstan!" "A line! A line! Give me a line there, for Davy Jones' sake!" and a great creaking of timbers. In the morning, there was the garden-seat, which was too big to float, dragged tilting into the pond, half in and half out.'

'*But you could put up with all this. How did the change come about?*'

'It was getting playful, obviously, and inventive, if ill-informed, and might have got dangerous. I decided to treat it with the consideration and dignity which it would probably later have insisted on, and I invited it in as a lodger, bedding it up in the old bathroom. At first I thought I would have to run canvas troughs up the stairs so it could get to its room without soaking the carpet, and I removed the flap from the letter-box so it would be free to come and go, but it soon learnt to keep its form quite well, and get about in macintosh and goloshes, opening doors with gloved fingers.'

'*Until a week ago . . .*'

'A week ago it started sitting with us in the lounge (and the electric fire had to be turned off, as

the windows kept on steaming up). It had
accidentally included a goldfish in its body, and
when the goggling dolt swam up the neck into the
crystal-clear head, it dipped its hand in and
fumbled about with many ripples and grimaces,
plucked it out, and offered the fish to my wife,
with a polite nod. She was just about to go into the
kitchen and cook the supper, but I explained
quickly that goldfish were bitter to eat, and he put
it back. However, I was going to give him a big
plate of ice-cubes, which he would have popped
into his head and enjoyed sucking, although his
real tipple is distilled water, while we watched
television, but he didn't seem to want anything. I
suppose he thinks he's big enough already.'

'*Free board and lodging, eh?*'

'I don't know what rent to charge him. I thought
I might ask him to join the river for a spell and
bring us back some of the money that abounds
there: purses lost overboard from pleasure-
steamers, rotting away in the mud, and so forth.
But he has grown very intolerant of dirt, and might
find it difficult to get clean again. Even worse, he
might not be able to free himself from his rough
dirty cousins, and come roaring back as an
impossible green seething giant, tall as the river
upended, buckling into the sky, and swamp us
and the whole village as well. I shudder to think
what would happen if he got as far as the sea, his
spiritual home: the country would be in danger. I
am at my wits' end, for he is idle, and lounges
about all day.'

'*Well, that's harmless enough . . .*'

'If he's not lounging, he toys with his shape,

restlessly. Stripping off his waterproof, he is a charming dolls'-house of glass, with doors and windows opening and shutting; a tree that thrusts up and fills the room; a terrifying shark-shape that darts about between the legs of the furniture, or lurks in the shadows of the room, gleaming in the light of the television-tube; a fountain that blooms without spilling a drop; or, and this image constantly recurs, a very small man with a very large head and streaming eyes, who gazes mournfully up at my wife (she takes no notice), and collapses suddenly into his tears with a sob and a gulp. Domestic, pastoral-phallic, maritime-ghastly, stately-gracious or grotesque-pathetic: he rings the changes on a gamut of moods, showing off, while I have to sit aside slumped in my armchair unable to compete, reflecting what feats he may be able to accomplish in due course with his body, what titillating shapes impose, what exaggerated parts deploy, under his macintosh. I dread the time (for it will come) when I shall arrive home unexpectedly early, and hear a sudden scuffle-away in the waste-pipes and find my wife ("just out of the shower, dear") with that moist look in her eyes, drying her hair: and then to hear him swaggering in from the garden drains, talking loudly about his day's excursion, as if nothing at all had been going on. For he learns greater charm each day, this Mr Waterman, and can be as stubborn as winter and gentle as the warm rains of spring.'

'I should say that you have a real problem there, but it's too early for a solution yet, until I know you better. Go away, take a week off from the office, spend

159

your time with your wife, relax, eat plenty of
nourishing meals, plenty of sex and sleep. Then come
and see me again. Good afternoon.

'The next patient, nurse. Ah, Mr Waterman. Sit
down, please. Does the gas fire trouble you? No? I can
turn it off if you wish. Well now, we're quite private
in here. You can tell me your troubles. A married, air-
breathing woman, I think you said. . . .'

Peter Redgrove

Slavewoman's Song

Ya howl –
Hear how ya howl –
Tell me wha ya howl foh
Tell me noh?
Pickni?
Dem tek pickni way?
Wha dem do wid pickni
Mek yu knaack yu head wid stone
Bite yu haan like daag-bone?

Is husban mek yu halla gal?
Wha dem do wid maan
Mek yu daub yu face wid cow dung
Juk yu eye an chap yu tongue?
Dem trow am Demerara, feed am alligita?

Muma? Pupa? Africa?
Belly big wid Massa?

Ya howl –
Hear how ya howl –
Tell me wha ya howl foh
Tell me noh?

David Dabydeen

Life/Death

Sudden,
Quick as light:
Skin shine,
Then
Bone white.

Ian McDonald

8.06 p.m. June 10th 1970

poem

Tom Raworth

Commentary

Well, last section. Doesn't time fly when you're
having fun? I've saved lots of the best until last:
poems that make people cross, poems that people
throw down in disgust, stamp on, set fire to and
then chuck the ashes in the canal because they're
not poems. Funny, isn't it, how some people
believe that certain kinds of poems shouldn't
exist?

Tom Leonard's 'A Summer's Day' is a love
poem, or rather a poem in which someone is
trying to declare something very close to love. Tom
Leonard is from Glasgow, and a number of his
poems are in this uncompromising language. I put
language and not *dialect*, because I think 'dialect'
can be a put-down. Why don't you have a go at
writing a poem in your own language? Don't tell
me you haven't got one. Invent one, if you like.

'Love Poem for Janet' is a performance poem by
a brilliant Welsh performance poet, Christopher
Mills. You've got to imagine it performed in Chris'
Cardiff accent, where it's all to do with the number
of a's. You've got to practise by saying "Caaardiff
Aaaarms Paaark." Try it at home in front of the
mirror. Performance poems are part of a long and
honourable (though not honoured) tradition that
goes back to the very roots of poetry, when people
accompanied their dancing by shouting. Have a go
at performing 'Love Poem for Janet'. It works well
with one voice, but you could try it with a number
of voices. How would it work with four voices?

'OK Gimme' by Martyn Wiley was jotted down in ten minutes at the side of a road in West Yorkshire. The poem can be sung as a round, with the 1st and 4th stanzas forming a backing chorus. It's since been performed by one, two, three, four and sometimes several hundred voices, which isn't bad for a list of things you say in New York if you're hungry.

'Trainspotter', by David Harmer and Martyn Wiley is a performance story poem. Tragic, isn't it?

There are found poems elsewhere in the book, but I can't resist dropping a couple more in. 'Country Dancing' by Peter Finch seems to me to be a pretty near perfect example of a found poem. The lines are just instructions from a dancing manual, but they make the poem seem to dance. 'The Holy Places' is a more considered piece, where Meg Peacock has had the luxury of being able to decide where to end the lines in the man's speech, and also by surrounding it by words of her own. It rhymes: I wonder if it's really a found poem, or did she alter the odd word to make it rhyme? Does it matter? Is it finders keepers?

One thing I never get tired of emphasising is that you don't have to understand a poem to enjoy it. You can like the sound of it, or the shape of it, or the images that are conjured up. One problem is that it's hard to describe to someone else what a poem that you don't understand does for you. '(Shades of Gone)' by Charlie Mehrhoff is one such poem. Charlie is an American Indian, but that knowledge doesn't help me to understand the poem.

'Mr Waterman' by Peter Redgrove isn't a poem, is it? I found it in a book of poems, so it must be a poem. But then that makes 'War and Peace' a poem, and my gas bill a poem. I once saw a man in a pub in Sheffield read his gas bill to a saxophone accompaniment. It was a huge gas bill.

I've tried to include lots of poems in languages other than standard English in this book, just to prove that you don't have to talk proper to write poetry. 'Slavewoman's Song' by David Dabydeen works wonderfully in Guyanese, but is a bit limp in the English translation. Ian McDonald is from Trinidad, and I put 'Life/Death' in because it's refreshing to have such a short poem with such a profound title. Speaking of short poems, '8.06 p.m. June 10th 1970' by Tom Raworth is the most profound and moving poem I've ever read. It beats anything else in the book by a mile.

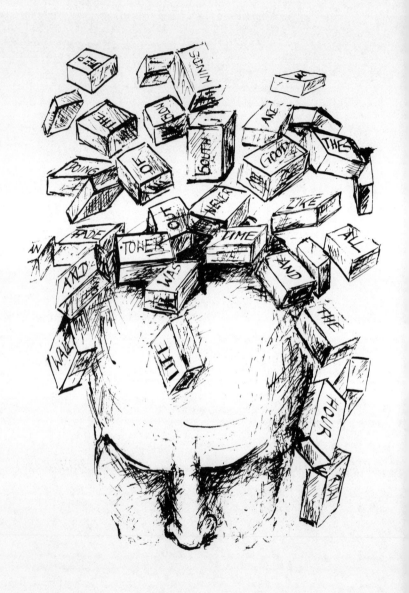

SECTION SIX

Things to do
- The Start of the World
- The Door
- The Apple
- Birthdays
- Birthdays and Baths

Where Do We Go From Here?
- Poetry Clubs
- Visiting Poets
- Days Out
- Publication

Address Hoard
- Regional Arts Associations
- Other Useful Addresses
- The Poetry Society
- The Arvon Foundation
- NAWE

Kake Yourself Comfortable   *Ian McMillan*

THINGS TO DO

The thing I want to emphasise here is that anyone
and everyone can write poems and stories. It's not
an odd thing to do, and you don't have to be a
special kind of person to do it. Everyone can do it.
You don't have to be in a poem-writing mood to
write poems, although it's true that if you're in a
certain mood it's easier to write certain kinds of
poems.

Try and make writing a normal, everyday and
enjoyable thing to do; keep a notebook of things
you see and things you hear other people say.
Keep a dream diary. Write down the view from
your window at 8.12am every day for two weeks,
and you'll have a fourteen-line beginning to a
poem. Build up a personal or classroom collection
of postcards: not just seaside postcards, but the
kind of postcards you get in art galleries or craft
shops. I've got a huge collection of these, and
I often use them to start my own writing off. You
could just describe a postcard, or you could
describe two contrasting postcards and then try
and find a way of linking them together. I'm very
keen on the idea of linking together, things that
seem to be apparently opposite. It's sometimes
worth getting two contrasting poems of your own
or of someone else's, and trying to make one
bigger poem out of the two.

I hope the poems in this book will give you
plenty of ideas for writing. On one level they
might make you want to write a poem about a

similar subject: the trio of grandma poems in section three might make you want to write a poem about your grandma, or about memories of your grandma.

You could also use the poems in a more practical way: borrow a title from a poem in the book and use it as a title for one of your poems. Take a first line, and then write a poem in which all the lines have the same rhythm as your first line. Then give the first line back (because you haven't really stolen it, you've only borrowed it), and invent a first line of your own. Or miss out the first line all together, and start with the second line, because I find that first lines are often redundant.

Often the hardest part of writing is getting started. Here are a few ideas to get you going. A lot of these exercises are examples of *guided fantasies*. In a way they're quite artificial exercises, but they often get you writing things you wouldn't normally write. And that's got to be a good thing.

The Start of the World

It's half an hour after the start of the world, and you're standing there, completely on your own, and you can't see anything. Just mist, grey mist. Then through the mist, three colours emerge. *Write them down*. They can be real colours or made-up colours. Then, you stand there looking at the colours and getting used to the idea of the world just consisting of colours, and then you hear three noises. What three noises do you think you might hear at the start of the world? *Write them down*. Then, through the mist you see two objects. One of them isn't a surprise; you expected to see it half an hour after the start of the world. The other object is a surprise. *Write down the two objects*.

Now, you're getting used to being on your own at the start of the world. Suddenly someone comes up behind you and taps you on the shoulder. Who could it be? It could be someone you know, or someone fictional. *Write down the name of the person*. You turn around and look at the person, and he or she says something to you. What would that person say to you? *Write it down*. Finally, the person taps you on the shoulder again, and points to something miles away, on the horizon: what could it be? *Write it down*.

You've now created a very strange world. Take one or two of the things, and use them as a starting point for a piece of writing.

The Door

Imagine a room from your childhood. It can be a public room, like a school room or a church room, or a private room in your house. Imagine the room as clearly as you can: the decoration, the furniture and so on. Then, imagine the door of the room: what kind of door is it. Then, someone knocks at the door. Who could it be? Perhaps it's someone from your childhood. You are in the room, and you go to the door and answer it. The person stands there, and gives you something. What could it be?

172

You give them something. What could it be? Think about this for a few minutes, and then *write down* your reactions to it. You'll often end up with a good basis for a poem.

The Apple

Imagine you've woken up in bed next to an apple. You're alone in the house, so how did it get there. *Write down how the apple got there.* You can write down scary, funny, or just silly reasons as to how the apple got there. After a while you decide to have a bite of the apple. There's something inside it: what could it be? *Write it down.* Anyway, you eat the whole apple, and it doesn't taste too bad, but then after an hour you turn into something. What could it be? *Write it down.*

Now, have a go at writing a three-stanza poem about the apple. Then substitute another word for the word 'apple'. I've used words like poem, story, song, star: "I woke up next to a star . . . I took a bite of it".

Birthdays

Write down the birth date of everyone in the room. Just the date will do, so in my case the 21st January would be 21. You'll end up with a list of random numbers. Now get a book, any book, but make sure that everyone in the room has got a different book. It doesn't really matter what kind of book it is: 'Five go off to the Canaries' is just as good in this context as 'War and Peace'.

Get the book and turn to the first page of actual text, missing out the contents and the printer's address and so on. If the first number on your list is 21, then write down the twenty-first word on the page. If the next number on the list is 7, then write down the seventh word after the 21st. Make your way down the page in this way. You'll end up with a list of random words, and the task is to make something from it. You often get startling and original poems from this exercise, which can stand very well as poems on their own, or which can be used as starting points for further work.

Birthdays and Baths

This is an extension of the previous idea. You get the list of words, as before, then, you imagine that you're having a bath. You're sitting in the bath and it starts to rain. It begins to rain heavier than it's ever rained before, and the earth begins to flood. The flood gets so bad that your house falls down, and you float out across the flood in your bath. It's frightening: you're all on your own (I hope!) and you've got nothing to eat or drink. You try to eat the soap but it makes you sick, and you try to eat the toy duck but it's a bit chewy. You can't drink the bathwater because it's all soapy and bath-foamy and horrible. You're starving and thirsty and frightened and cold and wet. You're tired, too, because you can't sleep: the only thing that's keeping the bath afloat is the plug. If the plug comes out, you're dead. So, you can't sleep because you're worried (in fact you're terrified) that the plug might come out.

But after thirty days and nights you're so exhausted that you fall asleep for twenty minutes. And you have a dream. What kind of dream would it be, bearing in mind that you're hungry and thirsty and all those other things? Think about the dream. *Now write the dream down*. No more than half a side of prose. Give yourself a one or two minute time limit.

Now, put your dream to one side. You wake up, and you've landed somewhere. An empty desert island. All of civilisation has been destroyed. All that's left of the whole of human knowledge is that bunch of random words. *Now make something from the words*.

Now, tear your dream up and put it in the waste bin. What a thing to do to a dream! When the whole group has torn their dream up, and put it in the bin, redistribute the dream to everyone. You might get a few bits of your own dream, but you'll mainly get bits of someone else's dream. If you get all your own dream back, write to me care of the publishers and I'll send you a prize. *Now make something from the dream fragments*

So, you'll end up with a mixture of beginnings, fragments, minimalist poems, and I can guarantee they'll be like nothing you've ever written before. Unless that's how you normally write your poems.

Variations on this kind of start are endless. Switch the radio on and off very quickly, then *write down the words you hear or what the music you hear reminds you of*, then use that as the first line/title/last line of a poem. Get someone to pass mystery objects around the room while you've all got your eyes shut, then, when you've opened your eyes, write down your reactions to feeling the object.

WHERE DO WE GO FROM HERE?

Okay, it's all very well doing these exercises and games, but how do you sustain the habit of writing poetry?

Poetry Clubs

Maybe your school could start a poetry club, meeting perhaps once a week or once a fortnight. I've been to lots of schools where they do this, and it's stimulating to get together and *enjoy* writing and reading and talking about poetry. The format of the club could vary. Some weeks you could read out and talk about your own poems, some weeks you could discuss your favourite poems, some weeks you could talk about poems you don't like and why you don't like them. An exciting part of the club could be that each week you write something together, either as a whole group or in pairs or groups of three, to get away from the idea that poems are things you write on your own.

They can be, but they don't have to be. Of course, teachers could start their own poetry club, or you could have a mixed teachers pupils poetry club. In fact, all the suggestions I'm making in this section are for teachers as much as for pupils.

Visiting Poets

This means you visiting the poet and the poet visiting you. A number of poets visit schools regularly. Organising a visit can be complicated, but it's often worthwhile.

First, choose your poet: either someone whose work you like, or someone who has been recommended to you by another school, or whatever. If you can't think who to invite, write to your local Regional Arts Association, and they'll suggest someone. There's a list at the back of the book. Once you've decided on your poet, write to him or her to see if they're free on the day you want them. Agree a mutual date and fee, and then apply to the Regional Arts Association, who will send you voluminous forms to fill in. The Regional Arts Association will usually then agree to subsidise part of the writer's fee. If you have any difficulty with any aspect of actually booking the writer, then speak to the Literature Officer at your Regional Arts Association and they'll be only too happy to help.

What you get the writer to do in your school is up to you. The writer can work with groups of selected pupils, with class size groups, or with larger groups: it's up to you and the individual writer to sort that out.

You could also visit the poet: keep an eye open for poetry readings taking place in your local library/arts centre/theatre or wherever. Check first that it's open for all ages and then get a school trip organised.

Days Out

Use your local environment as stimulation for poetry. Go out into the yard, go for a walk around the school, go for a walk to a specific place, and deliberately set out to make the trip a poem hunt. Take notes on what you see, write down words you see written down, and so on.

Art galleries are very good sources of poetic stimulation; lots of galleries have education officers these days, and they may well be able to provide you with workrooms as well as informed chat about the exhibits. I did a day-session once at Leeds City Art gallery with a group of pupils from John Smeaton High School, Leeds. We did a variation on the birthdays/shipwreck idea I described earlier, but we were able to use the sculptures as the things they found when they washed up. They wrote some wonderful poems! Other outdoor settings in which I've done poetry workshops – include a canal (with second year children near Runcorn), a castle, an outdoor sculpture park, a churchyard, a beach, and so on. The possibilities (as I keep saying) are endless.

Oh, and while you're out, find objects and take them back to school: you can make more poems from the objects!

An extension of the day out is the residential course. The Arvon Foundation runs two centres where schools can take parties for a week to work with professional writers; I can heartily recommend these as wonderful places to write poems. Again, the addresses are at the back. Maybe your school has a centre somewhere in the country: it would be worth having a poetry week there, sometime.

Publication

Once you've written the poems, why not publish them? If your school's got printing equipment, you can produce an anthology of the best work written during a week out, or the work produced during a day visit to a local museum, and then sell the booklet at a celebratory evening for parents and children, and use the profit to pay for a visit by a writer!

ADDRESS HOARD

Regional Arts Associations

Arts Council of Northern Ireland
181A Stranmillis Road
Belfast BT9 5DU
0232 663591

Eastern Arts
Cherry Hinton Hall
Cherry Hinton Road
Cambridge CB1 4DW
0223 215355

East Midlands Arts
Mountfields House
Forest Road
Loughborough
Leicestershire
LE11 3HU
0509 218292

Greater London Arts
9 White Lion Street
London N1 9PD
01 837 8808

Lincolnshire & Humberside Arts
St Hugh's
Newport
Lincoln
LN1 3DN
0522 33555

Merseyside Arts
Bluecoat Chambers
School Lane
Liverpool
L1 3BN
051 709 0671

Northern Arts
10 Osborne Terrace
Newcastle upon Tyne
NE2 1NZ
091 281 6334

North West Arts
12 Harter Street
Manchester
M1 6HY
061 228 3062

Southern Arts
19 Southgate Street
Winchester
Hampshire
SO23 9DQ
0962 55099

South East Arts
10 Mount Ephraim
Tunbridge Wells
Kent
TN4 8AS
0892 41666

South West Arts
Bradninch Place
Gandy Street
Exeter EX4 3LS
0392 218188

West Midlands Arts
Brunswick Terrace
Stafford
ST16 1BZ
021 631 3121

Yorkshire Arts
Glyde House
Glydegate
Bradford BD5 0BQ
0274 723051

Other Useful Addresses

Arts Council of Great Britain
105 Piccadilly
London W1V 0AU
01 629 9495

Literature Festivals Council
21 Earl's Court Square
London SW5 9DE
01 373 7861

National Community Folktale Centre
Middlesex Polytechnic
All Saints
White Hart Lane
London N17 8HR
01 801 3434

School Bookshop Association
1 Effingham Road
London SE12 8NZ
01 852 4953

The School Library Association
Liden Library
Barrington Close
Liden
Swindon SN3 6HF
0793 617838

Schools' Poetry Association
27 Pennington Close
Colden Common
Winchester
Hampshire SO21 1UR
0962 712062

The Poetry Society

The Poetry Society, funded by W. H. Smith, runs a
"Poets in Schools Scheme". For further details
write to: Education Officer
        The Poetry Society
        21 Earls Court Square, London SW5 9DE

The Arvon Foundation

Arvon has two centres which run five-day courses
with professional writers working alongside pupil
groups, student groups, teacher groups or
whatever.

Lumb Bank	Totleigh Barton
Hebden Bridge	Sheepwash
West Yorkshire	Beaworthy
HX7 6DF	Devon
	EX21 5ND

NAWE

The Northern Association of Writers in Education
seeks to bring together teachers and writers. It
puts on courses for writers and teachers and
produces a directory of writers who visit schools.
For further details contact:

NAWE
Irene Rawnsley
The Hollies
Stainforth
Settle
North Yorkshire

Acknowledgements

The author and the publishers wish to thank the following for permission to use copyright material:

Moira Andrew – 'My Father's Hands', 'Coming to Terms' and 'Tomorrow is Another Day', previously unpublished. **Simon Armitage** – 'And You Know What Thought Did' from *The Distance Between Two Stars*, 1987, The Wideskirt Press, Huddersfield. **John Ash** – 'A Novel' from *The Goodbyes*, Carcanet Press, Manchester. **Clive Benson** – 'I Used to Hate Andrew Lloyd Webber' from *Raw and Biting: Cabaret Poetry*, 1989 Pluto Press, London with Apples and Snakes, Covent Garden. **Val Bloom** – 'Mek Ah Ketch Har' from *Touch Mi Tell Mi*, Bogle L'Ouverture, London. **Gary Boswell** – 'Boiled Egg Deluxe', previously unpublished. **Alan Brownjohn** – 'In This City . . .' from *Alan Brownjohn: Collected Poems*, 1986, Secker and Warburg, London. **Jim Burns** – 'Social Poem' from *Poems for Tribune*, 1988, The Wideskirt Press, Huddersfield. **Duncan Bush** – 'Pneumoconiosis' from *Aquarium*, 1982; 'Cafe, Rainy Tuesday Morning' from *Salt*, 1985, Poetry Wales Press, Bridgend. **Terry Caffrey** – 'Scouse Apache', previously unpublished. **Charles Causley** – 'Forbidden Games' from *Poetry Society Compilation*, Poetry Society, London. **Gillian Clarke** – 'Cold Knap Lake' from *Poetry Book Society Anthology*, 1988, Hutchinson, London. **Paul Coltman** – 'Granny's Tale' from *Tog the Ribber (Granny's Tale)*, André Deutsch, London. **Tony Connor** – 'Grandma and the Blitz' from *New and Selected Poems by Tony Connor*, 1982, Anvil Poetry Press, London. **Stanley Cook** – 'The Dirty Man' from *New Poetry Two*, 1976, Arts Council, London. **Duncan Curry** – 'McCoy's Last Stand', previously unpublished. **Tony Curtis** – 'Strongman' from *Selected Poems*, 1986, Poetry Wales Press, Bridgend. **David Dabydeen** – 'Slavewoman's Song' from *Slavewoman's Song*, 1984, Dangaroo Press, Department of Caribbean Studies, University of Warwick. **Chris Darwin** – 'Grans' from *From the Heart of Liverpool 8*, 1984, Merseyside Worker Writers, Liverpool. **John Desmond** – 'Backwater', previously unpublished. **Maura Dooley** – 'Shadow on her Desk' from *Turbulence*, 1988, Giant Steps Press, Clapham, Lancaster. **Carol Ann Duffy** – 'Lizzie, Six' and 'A Healthy Meal' from

Standing Female Nude, 1985, Anvil Poetry Press, London; 'Mrs. Skinner, North Street' from *Neighbours*, Peterloo Poets, Calstock/BBC Publications, London. **Peter Finch** – 'Country Dancing' from *Selected Poems*, 1987, Poetry Wales Press, Bridgend. **Michael Gibbs** – 'Proverb (Tree Poem 4)' from *Typewriter Poems*, 1972, Second Aeon Publications, Cardiff. **Georgina Hammick** – 'Women on a Seaside Postcard, 1914' from *Poetry Book Society Supplement*, 1978, Poetry Book Society, London. **David Harmer** – 'Moose Malloy's First Poem' from *Spinner's Final Over*, 1982, Verse Wagon Press, Barnsley; 'Christmas Confessions' and 'Trainspotter', previously unpublished. **John Hegley** – 'Children' and 'Children with Adults' from *Raw and Biting: Cabaret Poetry*, 1984, Pluto Press, London with Apples and Snakes, Covent Garden. **Christine Herzberg** – 'Using Obscene Language', previously unpublished. **Jane Hollinson** – 'An Essay Justifying the Place of Science in the School Curriculum', from *Iron Magazine – Edition 56*, Iron Press, North Shields. **David Horner** – 'Like Strangers', previously unpublished. **Louise Hudson** – 'View from a Bus' from *Four Ways*, Phoenix Press, first published in *Smoke* magazine. **Robert Alan Jamieson** – 'Lion' from *Shormal*, Polygon, Edinburgh. **Stephen Knight** – 'The Gift' from *Introduction to Poetry, No. 6*, Faber and Faber, London. **John Latham** – 'From the Other Side of the Street' and 'Smoke Screen' from *From the Other Side of the Street*, 1986, Peterloo Poets, Calstock. **Tom Leonard** – 'A Summer's Day' from *Tom Leonard – Selected Poems*, 1986, Galloping Dog Press, Newcastle upon Tyne. **Liz Lochhead** – 'Everybody's Mother' from *True Confessions and New Clichés*, Polygon, Edinburgh. **Geoff Lowe** – 'Brombistle Bay' from *Proof*, 1987, Lincolnshire and Humberside Arts, Lincoln; 'How Do/Who Me', previously unpublished. **Sorley McLean** – 'Dogs and Wolves' from *Modern Scottish Gaelic Poems*, Canongate Publishing, Edinburgh. **Cavan MacCarthy** – 'Zeeeeyooosshhhhhhhh' from *Typewriter Poems*, 1971, Second Aeon Publishing, Cardiff. **Ian McDonald** – 'Life/Death' from *Mercy Ward*, 1988, Peterloo Poets, Calstock. **Charlie Mehrhoff** – '(Shades of Gone)' from *Psychopoetica Volume 12, Summer 1988*, Department of Psychology, University of Hull. **Christopher Mills** – 'Love Poem for Janet' from *Something's Awry*, 1988, Red Sharks Press, Cardiff. **Trevor Millum** – 'Birthdays', previously unpublished. **Edwin Morgan** – 'Wittgenstein on Egdon Heath' from *Poems of Thirty Years*, Carcanet Press, Manchester. **Paul Muldoon** – 'The Hands' from *Quoof*, Faber and Faber, London. **Grace Nichols** – 'Beauty' from *I is a Long Memoried Woman*, 1986, Virago Press, London. **Dorothy Nimmo** – 'A Woman's Work' from *Homeward*, Giant Steps Press, Clapham, Lancaster. **Alastair Paterson** – 'Danse Macabre' from *The Floating World*, 1984, Pig Press, Durham. **Meg Peacock** – 'Holy Places' from *Marginal Land*, 1988, Peterloo Poets, Calstock. **Tom Raworth** – '8.06 p.m. June 10th 1970' from *The Relationship*, 1969, Jonathan Cape, London. **Peter Reading** – 'An Everyday Story of Countryfolk' from *Fiction*, 1979, Secker and Warburg, London. **Peter Redgrove** – 'Mr Waterman' from *The Moon Disposes*, Secker and Warburg, London. **Alan Riddell** – 'The Honey Pot' from *Eclipse*, John Calder (Publishers) Ltd., London. **James Simmons** – 'A Birthday Poem' from *The Selected James Simmons*, Gallery Press, Dublin. **Martin Stannard** – 'Concerning "The Flat of the Land"' and 'The Ingredient' from *The Flat of the Land*, The Wideskirt Press, Huddersfield. **Janet Sutherland** – 'To the Spider in the Crevice Behind the Toilet Door' from *Dancing the Tightrope*, 1987, The Women's Press, London. **Leslie Ullman** – 'On Vacation a Woman Mistakes Her Leg' from *Natural Histories*, Yale University Press, New Haven, Connecticut, first published in *The New Yorker*, New York. **Jeffrey Wainwright** – 'The Migrant from England' from *Heart's Desire*, Carcanet Press, Manchester. **Martyn Wiley** – 'Singing in the Rain' and 'Admission' from *The Country Sundays*, 1986, Littlewood Press, Hebden Bridge; 'OK Gimme' and 'Trainspotter', previously unpublished. **Kit Wright** – 'Elizabeth', from *Bear Looked Over the Mountain*, Salamander Press. **Cliff Yates** – 'All Your Night', previously unpublished.

The author would also like to thank the following for their 'Against The Grain' poems: Shirley Bell, Iain Crichton Smith, Peter Finch, Arthur Kirby, Graham Mort, Lemn Sissay, Ken Smith

Kake Yourself Comfortable

Kome in. Sit Kown.
Kake yourself comfortable.

Kup of Kea? Bit of Kake?
Kilk? Kugar?

My problem? You Kish
to Kiscuss it?

Ah yes. The Ketter K.
Well, Kit all goes back

Ko Ky Khildhood. We were
very Koor. I only had one

Koy. A building Krick with
Ketters on. Except all the

Ketters Had Keen Kubbed off,
except one. All my childhood

I Konly Kever saw Kone letter.
The letter S.

Ian McMillan